THE ROAD TO
METABOLIC HEALTH

The Road to Metabolic Health

Why the Answer Lies in Food, Not Pharmaceuticals

Doug Reynolds, MHP

Published by Game Changer Publishing

Paperback ISBN: 978-1-965653-93-7

Hardcover ISBN: 978-1-965653-94-4

Digital ISBN: 978-1-965653-95-1

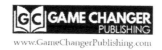

www.GameChangerPublishing.com

ACKNOWLEDGMENTS

Wow, I'm afraid to even start writing this because I know I am going to leave someone off here. If I do, please know that it is not intentional and I appreciate the contributions and help of absolutely everyone who has been part of our journey.

Obviously, first and foremost Pam Devine (my better half) who has been an integral part of creating and running both the organisations that we founded. I promised her that I wouldn't kill myself getting the book published before our event coming up in Boca next month, but she knew I would and I've even ended up killing her too, helping with the proofreading in order to make the deadline.

To Sarah Rice who has been a rock through all of this, who is responsible for most of what you will read about the ketogenic diet in Chapter 9, and who has kept me honest so that everything I have said is accurate.

To Tim Noakes and Gary Fettke for providing the shoulders for us all to stand on so that we can see further and to Gary, especially, for his mentorship and for being such a good friend.

And then to so, so many people who have influenced us, mentored us, supported us, worked alongside us, and helped us along the way: Belinda Fettke, Rod Taylor, Brian and Lanell Lenzkes, Rob and Janae Cywes, Dave Feldman and Sharon delPilar, Tro and Rosette Kalayjian, Dr Ben, Eric Westman, Mark Cucuzzella, Jodi Nishida,

Tia Reid, Karen Jerome-Zapdka, Vic Basmadjian, Evelyne Bourdua-Roy, Roxana Soetebeer, Andrea Salcedo, Bret Scher, Gurpreet Padda, Tony Hampton, Laura Buchanan, Matt Calkins (huge shoutout), Dom D'Agostino, Csilla Ari, Gary Taubes, Georgia Ede, Mike and Mary Dan Edes, Paul Mason, Eric Berg, Miriam Kalamian, Adrian Soto-Mota, Melanie Tidman, David and Judith Jehring, Sam Feltham, Campbell Murdoch, Olivia Khwaja, Susan Fairlie and the other folks at the PHC, Erin Bellamy, Jeff Gerber, Ivor Cummins, Peter Brukner, Pascal Lemieux, Beth McNally and Matt Miernik, Peter Ballerstedt, Jayne Bullen and Candice Spence and our other partners at the Nutrition Network, Nina Teicholz, Dave and Jen Unwin, Jeff Volek, Stephen Phinney, Tony Martinez, Adele Hite and Sarah Hallberg (both posthumously), Dorian Greenow and Gemma Kochis, Jennifer Isenhart and Tom Hadzor, Jeff and Tina Kotterman, Chris Cornell, to all the many speakers who have been on our stage, all our volunteers who have helped at so many events, all the attendees who have graced us with their presence at those events, and all those who don't come to mind as I feverishly write this up against the deadline, thank you is not sufficient!

More Resources

Just to say thank you for buying and reading my book,
I would like to refer you to some online resources to help you
on your journey to improved metabolic health. Scan the QR code
below for a list of resources where you can watch videos,
search for a practitioner, and print guidelines
for your doctor, among other useful information.

Scan the QR code for a list of resources:

https://bit.ly/the-road-to-metabolic-health

The Road to Metabolic Health

Why the Answer Lies in Food, Not Pharmaceuticals

Doug Reynolds, MHP

Disclaimer

The purpose of this work is to encourage the free exchange of ideas. The information in this document is not intended to replace a one-to-one relationship with a qualified healthcare professional and should not be considered medical advice. It is presented as a sharing of knowledge and information derived from the research and experiences of the authors of this document, as well as those of the numerous cited papers, books, and websites. The author encourages you to make your own healthcare decisions based on your research and in collaboration with a qualified healthcare professional.

The statements made in this document have not been evaluated by the FDA (US Food and Drug Administration). Any information published herein is not intended to diagnose, treat, cure, or prevent any disease. It is not a substitute for an in-person consultation with your doctor and should not be construed as individual medical advice.

FOREWORD

It is one thing to try and make a change. It is another to do it. Herding healthcare professionals to a cause requires a passion. Doug's 'low-carb' journey has not been travelled for himself, but for you and for us all.

Over time, I have come to realise that Doug and I have had similar influences that shaped us into who we are today, and to what we aim to achieve.

We both have southern African backgrounds – Doug directly and me through family history.

I have both played sport with and against South African sportsmen. They are tough but fair, competitive until the end, and leave their aggression on the field. A good feed, drink and yarn to follow, and you realise we have more in common than not. Doug and I have both had major head traumas that we have largely recovered from. Mine was in surgical management of a tumour, and Doug's was purely traumatic. There is something very personal with a head injury and the recovery. You need massive family support and personal drive through the foggy times, the self-doubts and the long recovery – you need a degree of grit.

For me, and I believe also for Doug, it made me aware of my mortality, my vulnerability, and the short time that I have on this planet. It gives you drive, passion and a degree of impatience to achieve something meaningful, damning the personal consequences at times. You will find a lot of these characteristics in Doug's story. The combination of grit, drive, passion, impatience and personal commitment are all there in this story of the formation of LowCarb*USA* and The Society of Metabolic Health Practitioners.

One of the major career turning points for me, as both a surgeon and as a patient, was the realisation that we are surrounded by metabolic health issues from birth to death. These are lifestyle-related complications and require lifestyle-related management – the answer is not in medicating our way out of these problems. The answer is simple in *The Road to Metabolic Health*. Returning to our evolutionary ways of eating and exercising.

———

Doug fondly tells the story of him and Pam visiting Belinda and me in Tasmania several years ago. I'm still trying to remember if we invited them to stay or they gate crashed in. Most people do not recover from a weekend of information overload from us both. 'Conspiracies' and 'fad' diets are neither when they are based on fact and science. At the end of that weekend, Doug and Pam became great friends as well as carrying another layer of insight forward to a wider community. We made our way to San Diego the following year to support the LowCarb*USA* event and we remain supporting each other's journey from opposite sides of the world. Once you realise you are part of a community, making a change across the world, then a few time zones are nothing in this connected world.

Our low-carb friends, near and far, past, present and future, are making a difference. We are on the same team. We are all playing our individual roles but part of a greater movement to empowering the health of ourselves, our children and our wider community. Therapeutic Carbohydrate Restriction is becoming best practice management in guidelines. We might have had to write them ourselves in recent times, but they are gaining recognition and institutional adoption. It's good to be on the winning team.

The Road to Metabolic Health is equally education and inspiration. You will find a bit of both in there for you.

– Dr Gary Fettke
Orthopaedic Surgeon, Tasmania, Australia
M.B.,B.S.(University NSW), F.R.A.C.S.
(Orthopaedic Surgery), F.A.Orth.A., MHP

CONTENTS

·

INTRODUCTION

My name is Doug Reynolds. I am an electrical engineer by training, but during my early years, I evolved into the role of a software engineer.

A lot has happened in my life since then, and currently, I run two organisations. One is called LowCarb*USA*®, which offers support and training for practitioners and patients – particularly for those whose doctors are unwilling, or don't know how, to help them – adopt Therapeutic Carbohydrate Reduction (TCR), a strict version of which is commonly known as the ketogenic diet, to manage many of the chronic conditions prevalent in today's society. Over the years, as part of that effort, a nonprofit group called the Society of Metabolic Health Practitioners (SMHP™) came about. This organisation is for all practitioners who embrace – or are considering – this therapeutic intervention and practise metabolic medicine, raising awareness and educating and providing ongoing support for them. We provide them with all the training they need to earn accreditation, and the growing consensus amongst all these practitioners will lead to the establishment of an alternative Standard of Care (SoC) so that practitioners can feel supported, too.

I am the CEO of LowCarb*USA* and the President of the SMHP. I have often thought to myself, *How the hell did I get here? I trained as a software engineer. What am I doing helping to educate healthcare practitioners about reducing carbohydrates in their patients' diets in order to help them reverse conditions like type 2 diabetes and to address numerous other chronic conditions, including neurological ones like Alzheimer's and Parkinson's, and even many mental health conditions?*

All these chronic conditions that we suffer with as a society can be shown, as we'll see later in the book, to be fundamentally attributed to insulin resistance caused by chronic excessive carbohydrate consumption, as Dr Robert Cywes puts it. But yeah, how did I get here? How did that even happen? I've often thought about it and mentioned to Pam and several other people that I feel like I've had a very interesting life, going all the way back to being born in Rhodesia (now Zimbabwe), and that there was probably a book in there somewhere.

I just wanted to write this book so that people could get to know me better. Some of the experiences I had growing up were just not what the average person, especially here in the United States, would have been exposed to. Throughout my life, there were so many things I attempted – like trying to start many projects and businesses – that failed, but it feels like every single thing that I went through from back when I was a little kid, right up until the time that I decided to start LowCarb*USA,* was preparing me for that moment. I felt like people might be interested in knowing how this all started.

At LowCarb*USA*, we hold conferences and bring in scientists and medical practitioners to teach about the science and benefits of carbohydrate reduction. During my opening talk at each of the events, I start out by introducing myself and telling the story about how LowCarb*USA* came to be and eventually the SMHP too. I only have a few minutes to speak, so the story always starts from when I first heard about the ketogenic diet and what a profound effect it had on me and concludes with how it finally led up to the decision to pull the trigger and go and put on the first conference that started this whole thing.

I have told this story so many times at the events (we've done 22 now) and during numerous podcast interviews that Pam often says to me, 'You always tell the same story.'

I know what she means, but my answer is always, 'Well, that's because that's the story. I don't want to make anything up.'

But now, in this book, you can read the *whole* story. You'll learn about everything that prepared me for, and everything that led up to, my making the decision to put on that first event in San Diego. And then there's all the drama leading up to those first few events – issues no one's even heard of – that will make you think it's a miracle we're still here!

Over the years, we have developed a tribe, a community of people, practitioners, and patients who want to learn about metabolic medicine. It's been growing organically but slowly. We've been able to help so many people, and many of these people are able to reach and teach others. We know that there are so many more people out there who are very sick and need our help, but we don't reach them. They're not within our sphere of influence, our social media presence, or our newsletter list that people opt into. I feel like the majority of the people who really need help are beyond our reach.

We are constantly looking for ways to reach more people, burst out of our bubble, and reach beyond that. It's so important that we get to more people, and my hope is that we will be able to achieve some of that through the publication of this book. I hope this book, which shares my journey and the changes that inspired me to start an organisation to help others, will keep readers (like you) engaged. Through my story, you'll learn how metabolic medicine, along with lifestyle and dietary changes, can drastically improve – and even save – lives. Then, they can learn about the organisations we have put in place to help them achieve that. If you finish this book feeling like there is so much more you need to learn, then I've done my job.

So, let's go back to my early days, growing up in Rhodesia, and I will tell you how I believe those experiences helped develop my character and a belief in myself that I could do anything I set my mind to. In fact, if something needs to be done, backing down because it is dangerous or risky doesn't even occur to me.

CHAPTER 1

THE EARLY YEARS

My dad was born in Sarawak, Borneo, which was a British colony in those days. Head-hunting was a common practice in Borneo back in the early 1900s, but by the time my dad was born in 1930, the practice had been brought to an end. As the commissioner of police there, his father would have had a hand in bringing that about. I'm not sure that it has much to do with why I'm here doing what I'm doing today, but it's a cool story! When my dad was still very young, the family moved to South Africa, and he went to school in Cape Town. When he finished high school, he wanted to be a farmer, but there weren't really any opportunities in South Africa for him to do that.

However, Southern Rhodesia (which became Rhodesia and then Zimbabwe) was just to the north, and there were opportunities there as a lot of farmers were looking to hire farm managers. But he didn't have a job as a farm manager yet and so for his immigration application to move up there, he applied to join the police force.

He moved to Salisbury (now Harare), Southern Rhodesia, and became a policeman. His plan was to serve out the minimum number of years he was required to commit to when he joined and then go find a job as a farm manager.

But it turns out that he was an extremely good rugby player, and he made it into the Southern Rhodesian national side in pretty short order. So he was playing rugby for the police club team and then playing for the national side as needed. That became a huge part of his life, so he stayed where he was and was still serving in the police and playing rugby nine years later.

One day, as he was training, he put his neck out while practising his kicking. The injury ended his rugby career. I'm pretty sure a good chiropractor would have had him back on the field the next day, but they knew nothing of that back then, and he still doesn't believe in chiropractors to this day. Now, suddenly, he was looking at his life and thinking, *Well, I came up here to become a farmer. Maybe this was meant to be, so now I need to go farming.*

So that is what he did. He found a job as a manager on a farm. He had a couple of managing positions on different farms and was able to learn the job along the way. After a while, he was offered an opportunity on a massive farm where the plan was that he would work as the manager for a while, and at some point, there would be a division. The owner was actually going to divide the land, and my dad would have the opportunity to acquire ownership of his own farm.

But the whole thing fell apart. I've never really been able to get to the bottom of what happened, but he came back into town with the idea that he was going to look for another opportunity.

However, until another opportunity came up, he needed to earn some money. I hate smoking so much that I don't like to bring it up, but a lot of what the farmers grew there was tobacco. Once the tobacco has been grown, harvested, cured, and baled, it gets shipped into town to be auctioned. Different cigarette companies would send buyers to 'the floors' to purchase the tobacco based on whether it was the grade that they were looking for. My dad was actually one of those buyers.

The auction itself was quite a process, with all the bales being laid out in long lines and all opened up so that the buyers could inspect the grade of the tobacco in each one. The line of buyers would move ahead of the auctioneer and be between two and ten bales ahead of him. So they would be inspecting the grade of one bale while bidding on the purchase of one they looked at a few bales back and even bidding on ones they didn't want just to push up the prices for their competitors.

I suppose the same sort of thing happened for him here as it did in the police force. No great farming offers came along, so he just kind of stayed where he was. I don't think he felt like he could afford to just go and buy a farm. It would have to be a similar deal to the one he had had before. In the end, he never got back out farming again.

It was around that time that I came along. We lived in Salisbury. We were basically an average blue-collar family, but the lifestyle there was quite privileged. We lived in a really nice house on an acre of land with a swimming pool, and everybody had live-in domestic workers. We had a gardener and a domestic worker, but he didn't just clean the house; he was a really good cook, too. Everything we ate back then was home-cooked real food, no processed food in sight.

When I think back on it, the lifestyle was also very active. Rugby and cricket were the national sports, and they were massively popular. Most kids at school played one of those sports, and there was tennis and netball for the girls (girls didn't play rugby back then) in the winter and athletics and cross country during the summer. Pretty much everyone participated in something athletic; very few didn't.

There were no computer games either. When we used to visit our friends, we would run around and play cops and robbers and other games like that. We'd run around like crazy kids in the garden (which was always at least an acre of land). Running around chasing each other, we ended up running for miles.

It was very healthy from that perspective. And the food we ate was the way that grandma used to prepare food – real, whole food.

Mom would go and buy different types of meat: pork, chicken, beef, and all the different cuts of meat that she would be planning for the various menus throughout the week. We ate meat and vegetables every day. And that was just normal. I remember her having this little enamel dish in the fridge. I was, I don't know, six years old, maybe, but I have this vision of her pouring the rendered fat from her cooking through a filter into that dish and letting it harden in the fridge.

When she wanted to cook something like burgers in the frying pan, she would get a spatula and gouge a whole lump of this fat out of the dish, chuck it in the pan, and start cooking with it. That's such a vivid memory for me. I don't know why, but it's something that I can literally see her doing right now as I'm talking about it.

The milk was fresh, too. It was delivered by a guy who drove around in a truck and basically came and brought your order to the house: two, three, four, or six bottles of milk each day. It would be in these glass bottles with this big, thick head of cream at the top of each bottle that had settled out of it. Really, full cream milk in the true sense of the word. And I think those deliveries were coming directly from some farm just out of town for sure. I loved it, but fast forward a few years, and that would all disappear.

What we ate back then is very different from what's being advocated these days by the US dietary guidelines. I don't know if being exposed to that when I was young made me more open to acknowledging down the road that eating all the rubbish advocated in the dietary guidelines was maybe not such a good thing. Maybe eliminating processed food and excessive carbohydrates and going back to eating real food just made sense.

Since my dad had been farming, he had a lot of friends who were farmers. We used to go out during our school holidays (vacations) and spend time with those friends on the different farms. I just loved it, as most kids would, I suppose. On one of the farms we used to visit on weekends or for a few days at a time, I must have been seven or eight (maybe) – there were these tractors everywhere. I didn't get involved in ploughing, or anything like that, but there was a service tractor that used to have a big trailer attached to the back that they would take workers and other supplies out to the fields. Taking salt blocks out to put out in the pastures for the cattle to lick on was a regular trip. I was really small, but I would go and speak to the tractor driver and tell him I wanted to drive his tractor. He showed me how to do it, and then, as this tiny little kid, I was driving a tractor and trailer around the farm, often with a bunch of workers on the trailer behind me. The driver would literally sit on the hubcap of the tractor next to me so that he could help me if I ever ran into trouble, which I didn't ever, by the way. Being able to drive something that big and feel that important when I was so young was so cool and always really exciting. It didn't matter what time they were going out. Even at four o'clock in the morning, I was there, and I was going to drive. So, for the whole time we were there, I would drive the tractor whenever it needed to go somewhere. I'm sure the regular driver was glad to see the back of me when we returned to town.

There were other farms we visited where the farmers had kids, and on one of them in particular, they had a son called Robbie, who was the same age as me. From about the age of 10–13, we would go out and visit for the weekend at the beginning of the school holidays and then when my folks went back to town to return to work, I would stay behind, and that was a whole different experience.

So the big thing at that time was that there was a guerrilla war going on. It never really infiltrated the cities (as it would later in South Africa), so pretty much all the attacks that occurred were happening out on the open roads outside of the towns and cities and on the farms.

It was the farmers and the people travelling outside of the city who were always at risk. I remember that the farmhouses had grenade screens over the windows so that these guerillas couldn't lob grenades into the house from the garden. During that time security fences also started to go up around the homesteads that hadn't been there in the early years when I first used to visit these farms.

All the farms had a system installed called Agri-Alert, which connected them to the rural police station. Anytime there was an incident, a farmer could jump on there and report what was going on so the police could send help. Each farm also had to check in at a certain time every morning and night, almost like a roll call. If one of the farmers didn't call in, then the police would send people out to see if they were okay. I remember us all sitting around waiting for our turn to check in and hoping no one missed.

It didn't stop life from carrying on, though. One of the really vivid memories and stories that I have from back then was when Robbie's father used to go out into the lands really early in the morning to oversee the ploughing or whatever else was going on in the fields.

We would eat breakfast after he left, and then his mom would pack a picnic basket with breakfast for us to take to him. They had this little Honda 90, like a little moped or motorbike we would use to do this. Like with the tractor, kids love to get to drive something, so this was huge. We would both ride on the scooter, and whoever got to drive going out, the other guy got to drive coming back.

Whoever wasn't driving would sit on the back with the breakfast basket on his lap. And on top of that was, if I remember correctly, an old World War II Sterling submachine gun. It's basically like an Uzi-type machine gun with a 34-round magazine, and there was a spare magazine in the basket with the breakfast, too.

And literally, as 10-, 11-, 12-, or 13-year-old kids, we would drive around like that, and it was normal. Not only that, my parents let me go there and be a part of this. They would drop me off at the farm, and then they pick me up two or three weeks later, as the holidays were ending. They took me there, knowing full well what the situation was, and yet they were happy to drop me off. I think, if I look back, maybe that's where my not letting fear prevent me from doing something came from. I think that is what came out of that for me: When something is risky, or I have some kind of fear about it, that doesn't factor into the decision to do it if it really needs to be done.

One of the other things that I think helped a lot was that I became involved with the Boy Scouts. I was involved with this movement for my entire time there until I was 14, when we moved to South Africa. In the early years, it was the Cubs, and then, as I got older, I moved up to the Scouts.

I feel like two things impacted me the most. First of all, Friday evenings were when we would have our meetings. The clubhouse was in the middle of nowhere in an area with just bushes all around it – there were no houses anywhere nearby. It was nighttime, so it was dark, and we would play these games. One of the games that we used to play, I remember, was called 'Hunt the Lantern.' We used to break up into two groups, and one group would have a lantern, which they had to keep on at all times. They would go off into the bushes to hide it or conceal it as best as possible and then try to defend it. Everyone else was a stalker, and we would each have a scarf tucked into and hanging out of our pants. If a defender got your scarf, you had to go back to the clubhouse. So we were running around in the pitch dark, literally, in the bush. With the things that go on in society nowadays, I'm not sure those sorts of games would not be allowed to happen anymore.

The part I enjoyed most, however, was an activity called 'pioneering'. They had this huge pile of telephone poles and boxes of ropes of all different lengths and diameters in the shed at the back, and we would be set tasks to build things like platforms and bridges to get us across a ravine or a river, or to create a *foefie slide* (zip line) and other cool things. They taught us all the lashings and knots we needed to know to make the structures really sturdy, and then they let us loose to design and come up with whatever we were tasked with. I think the ingenuity and out-of-the-box thinking that these activities cultivated in us was priceless. It made me believe that any problem could be solved, I suppose. Put your head down and think about it, and you'll come up with a solution. I believe that all those experiences were formative, preparing me to make that decision one day to do something important and find a way to make it happen.

Sports in school were pretty much compulsory. Everybody had to do something. And not only that, but you needed to be there to support the senior teams when they played as well. My last few years in Rhodesia were my first two and a half years of high school, so I was a junior in the school. They don't have the concept of freshman, sophomore, junior, and senior there. High school was five years and even six if you went on to do your A-Levels. Sports practice was in the afternoon during the week, but matches were on Saturdays. As juniors, our teams were sometimes scheduled in the mornings. We would need to take our opposing number from the visiting team home for lunch and then bring him back in the afternoon to watch the senior games. Everyone in attendance from the visiting school would be seated in the grandstands, and the entire school from the home team would be on stands (bleachers) on the other side that ran almost the whole length of the pitch. If your game was after lunch, then you were allowed to be there in your school tracksuit, but the rest of us were in full school uniforms, blazers and all.

We all had to learn a bunch of war cries and chants, and a few of the seniors would parade along in front of the stands and lead the war cries. The sound was really impressive, and we were so proud to be a part of it.

At first, I grumbled a bit about the attendance being compulsory and it taking up our whole Saturday. But after that first home game, the feeling of camaraderie and pride was incredible, and I never complained again. I was just so proud to be a part of that school. Later on, this understanding of how important it is for people to be a part of, and proud of, something would result in me putting so much effort into cultivating and nurturing our community.

When I was 14, my parents decided that they were going to move down to South Africa. I mentioned earlier that a lot of the attacks would happen on either the farms or the rural roads. The busiest road out of Salisbury was the one going all the way down to Beitbridge, which was on the South African Border. It was also where the most attacks occurred. In order to try to minimise the attacks, the army set up this convoy system. They had a staging post right outside Salisbury where everyone would meet early in the morning, and they created these vehicles – I believe in the military here in the States, they call them 'technicals'. But they basically built these things with a bakkie (pronounced 'bucky', also called a pickup truck in the US and a 'ute' in Australia). They mounted a gun turret in the bed of the truck that could swing around 360 degrees, and it had armour plating in front to protect the gunner.

They would have one at the back and one at the front. And then, every ten cars or so, they would have one of these modified bakkies with a machine gun on it. And so this big procession would drive down to the South African border each day. Once they started doing that, it actually prevented any further attacks from happening, but they were still occurring on all the other roads where this kind of support didn't exist. Just normal life!

CHAPTER 2

A New Life in South Africa

Once we crossed the Limpopo River into South Africa, however, everything changed. More often than not, you don't have a clue what sort of stress you are living with until it's not there anymore. For now, the stress was gone, and it was very noticeable, even to me as a kid – but after some time, things would escalate in South Africa as well. For now, we were headed to a place called the Vaal Racecourse.

Just as my dad had to join the police force in order to have a job that he was moving to when he immigrated to Rhodesia, moving down to South Africa was the same thing. You couldn't just pitch up there and say, 'Hey, I'm coming to stay.' You had to have a job offer in your hands to do that.

So he had been a farmer, and a policeman, and he had worked as the starter at the Borrowdale Racecourse in Salisbury. Managing the racecourse is basically like all those jobs in one. You've got this massive property, and the racecourses in South Africa are all grass. They have sand tracks on the inside of the course for training, but the racing was on this massive grass track. It was about 3.2 kilometres around – roughly two miles – and approximately 50 metres wide.

There was all this thick Kikuyu grass that made up the track that needed to be continuously mowed and managed. A huge amount of land around it had to be maintained, along with the grandstands. Then we had roughly 500 horses on the property as well, so there were all those stables and all the grooms for all those horses. 500 grooms lived in a hostel on the property, and all my dad's workers for the racecourse itself also had their own hostel.

He was managing all of that, and there was often a lot of drinking and fighting going on in the hostels, which he also had to deal with. His police and farming experience made him the perfect candidate to manage this place. He had been working as a handler and a starter at the horse races on Saturdays back in Salisbury, so he had actual knowledge of the racing scene as well, which also helped. We moved down there, about an hour's drive south of Johannesburg (known colloquially as Joburg) in the Vaal Triangle. There were towns in that area called Vereeniging, Sasolbug, and Vanderbijlpark (fun-der-bile-park), and that was the Vaal Triangle, which literally made a triangle on the map.

Right in the centre of that triangle was this little coal mining town called Viljoensdrif (fill-you-ens-drif), and a kilometre down the road from there was the racecourse, it was literally like a farm. There were no other properties around; there was my dad's home, his assistant's home, and the security guy lived on the property as well. But it was like three homesteads on a farm. I had lived in town as a kid and spent as much time as I could on a farm. Now I lived on a racecourse, and for me as a kid, it was just like living on a farm.

So there was a coal mine and a power station a bit further down the main road from the racecourse. It was about a mile that we would have to go up this little road to get up to the main road, which went directly into town. There was a school bus that came in from the coal mine and power station, which brought all the kids into town for school. We would stand out on this main road, literally across the road from the Viljoensdrif station. It was just a station and a little deli-type shop on the platform and an exchange, like a manual tele-phone exchange with three operators who worked there – Willie, Magda, and Mara.

We literally had this phone with a little handle on the side, and you'd have to spin the handle to contact the operator. Then the oper-ator on the exchange, Willie, Magda or Mara, would say, 'Nommer asseblief? (Number please?)' and you'd tell them what city and number you wanted. They would put it through for you (and often listen in on the calls) like you see in the movies back in the olden days. If somebody else wanted to call our phone number from outside, they would have to call the main national exchange and ask for Viljoensdrif 1-5 – that was our number, Viljoensdrif 1-5!

Anyway, the bus stop was not really a stop but just a place where the bus could pull off the road. We used to stand there and wait for the school bus in the mornings, and in the winter, it was freezing (for us). I remember -12° Celsius (10° Fahrenheit) being typical. I think -16° (3° Fahrenheit) was the coldest I ever remember seeing. We had a thermometer outside our kitchen door, and it was the first thing we looked at as we walked out the back door each morning to go to my dad's bakkie that he would take us up to the bus stop in.

And we would stand up there with these huge trucks coming from the coal mines that would come barreling past. And when it was already -12°, the wind from those vehicles made it really tough. There we were, the three of us – my brother, my sister, and me – absolutely freezing while waiting for the bus.

On the way up to the bus stop in the mornings, my sister and I used to sit on the bench seat in the front of the bakkie with my dad. Because my brother was the youngest, he had to go in the back. To this day, I've got visions of him cowering against the back of the cab of the bakkie, trying to get out of the wind in this freezing cold weather. He never once complained; he never asked why he had to be the one to go in the back. I think I would have complained. It wasn't fair; we should have taken turns or something. I would never have tolerated being the only one to sit in the back every day, all the way through winter.

That's just a fun little story, but getting into this new school was a big shock. I mentioned earlier that, suddenly, there wasn't that same pride in belonging to that school. It was just like a pain in the butt to have to be there. You went to your classes, and you came home, and that was it. No one really had pride in being a part of that school, representing it or trying to play a sport for it.

We arrived in South Africa when it was about six weeks before the end of that school year. Primary school in South Africa was the first seven years, KG1, KG2, then Standard 1 to 5. Then high school (senior school) was five years from Standard 6 to 10. My brother and sister were still in primary school when we arrived, and that was literally next door to the high school. It was a very different culture, I had to finish out Standard 7 at the high school on my own.

I struggled a bit with that, but in the new year, I went into Standard 8 and my sister came through to start high school, so she went into Standard 6.

The school was divided up into four houses and early in the year, we had this inter-house athletics competition where all the students from each of the different houses competed against each other. All the participants who placed in the top 3 in each event qualified for the inter-high team, which then competed against other high schools in the area.

It was announced at the assembly in the morning that there was going to be practice for the inter-high school athletics team. My sister and I showed up after lunch like we were expected to; I mean, obviously we're going to go to show up for practice, right? But it was me, my sister, and the head girl of the school at the time who were the only three people who showed up. And that was a real shock to us.

It felt weird, too; we weren't comfortable at all. We really felt like we had to lean on each other for support through those times because there was a lot of bullying going on. We suffered with that bit, but it was just because we were different, I suppose. The first day at the school, I showed up in my grey school shorts from Rhodesia and was unmercifully ridiculed because 'you only wear long grey trousers at high school'. It took a while for us to feel like we were a part of that school.

Then at the end of Standard 8. We got a new headmaster, Mr Staples, and he was very different. I think he saw the same thing that we saw, and he believed that kids needed to belong to something and feel proud of that.

So he started to make inter-high team practice – and even practices for the inter-house competition – compulsory. I vividly remember attending the inter-high athletics meeting during my Matric year (equivalent to Standard 10, our final year of high school). It was amazing to see not only the students competing but also a group of students who came, of their own volition, purely to support the team and show school spirit. The new headmaster did that in two years, and it was an enormous feat. It was awesome to feel proud of being a part of something again, and this would continue on into my years at university and beyond.

As you'll see later, our LowCarb*USA* launch started out as a simple event but swiftly expanded into something much more. Early on, I recognised the need to establish a community to support the professionals and patients implementing TCR or, in the strictest sense, the ketogenic diet, as a means of addressing long-term health concerns (you'll learn more about that later also). Because the medical establishment did not consider this intervention to be Standard of Care, these people were frequently criticised and ostracised. For many, the journey was extremely difficult because they were on their own.

Thinking back on my own school and college experiences, I recalled the significance of feeling a sense of belonging and that memory inspired me to make LowCarb*USA* more than just a series of events. My goal was to establish a 'home' where patients and practitioners could interact, exchange stories, discuss cases, and compare notes. It surprised us at first, but many connect and plan future work together, collaborations for future conversations, partnership in practices and, or research projects. This sense of community serves as the cornerstone of our work and we continue to work on cultivating it as best we can.

Meanwhile, I can't help but reflect on my early years and how our family's life was impacted by dietary changes. During my high school years in South Africa, I saw the demonisation of saturated fat, like butter and animal fat, as well as the rise of the low-fat dietary guidelines. The way that families, including mine, prepared meals was significantly impacted by these changes. Margarine and seed oils took the place of butter and saturated fats, and even the milk in our refrigerator was replaced with skim milk. I can still clearly recall how terrible skim milk tasted – so bad that it broke my habit of snatching sips directly from the bottle, which used to annoy my mother!

It's a fact that your body knows what it wants. As humans evolved over time, we understood what our bodies needed, and the hunter/gatherers would go out and get what they needed. We subconsciously figured out what our bodies needed to eat. Once we started introducing agriculture and cutting saturated fat out of everything and adding vegetable oils and processed foods, we started to become less healthy. Seed oils are the most ultra-processed ingredients out there. Butter and cream are natural but they were being excluded from our diet. Over the years, that affected me and by the time I was 50 and I learned about the ketogenic diet, I was 35 pounds overweight with all sorts of inflammatory and respiratory issues.

It doesn't happen overnight. It's not like a switch, where you start eating this rubbish, and the next day you start developing problems. Rather, it's a chronic thing that creeps up on you, and before you know it you're really unhealthy. You will probably just attribute it to getting older but from what I have experienced, that's not the case. It's not about getting old; it's about just living an unhealthy lifestyle for so long that it finally catches up with you. I think the most amazing thing that I discovered was that a lot of it can be reversible, even at an older age. Of course, there are certain neurological conditions like Alzheimer's that, once they start developing, are really difficult, if not impossible, to reverse. But we're seeing there are stages where symptoms can be altered drastically by adding good, natural fats and good sources of nutrients, proteins especially.

Autism in children is another big one that may be preventable if they are brought up to eat properly from infancy. There's an Australian movie called *The Magic Pill* that showed a couple of examples of autistic children who were positively affected by taking all the carbohydrates and processed food out of their diets. They began eating real food again and their autism symptoms improved substantially, although they were never able to get back to 100%. Some of the damage was permanent.

However, there seem to be all sorts of things that are pretty much reversible if you change what you eat and fix your lifestyle, like type 2 diabetes. It's kind of amazing how things can be reversed just by eating what Dr Ken Berry likes to call the Proper Human Diet. Of course, exercise is important too and kids naturally get lots of it if they are being active and playing sports.

Over the years, I focused on endurance sports like ultramarathon running. I became extremely fit as a result of that training, but I later discovered that exercise is more than just cardio. After we established LowCarb*USA,* we were approached by Dr Ben Bocchicchio, a pioneer in muscle health and fitness. I received a direct message from Dr Ben, who insisted he should be speaking at one of our conferences. I initially offered him a breakout session during lunch rather than a main stage talk. I did not have time to attend his talk, but I was shocked to learn how well his session went – he sold out of more than 100 books in minutes! He became a regular at our events and was a keynote speaker by the following year. He has a unique perspective on high-intensity exercise, and my mind has changed completely since meeting him. You'll learn a lot more about Dr Ben later.

When I reflect on the past 40 years, I can see how our health has been weakened by misguided dietary and lifestyle recommendations.

I have personally witnessed how much of this damage can be undone by adopting healthier eating and lifestyle habits.

As we proceed, I will go into greater detail about these ideas and how community can help this life-changing experience. For the time being, though, let us move on from high school to university and the lessons there that helped to shape my future.

CHAPTER 3

THE UNIVERSITY YEARS

After high school, I went to the University of the Witwatersrand (Wits, pronounced 'Vits') in Joburg and began to study electrical engineering.

Now, my parents could never afford to send me to university. The only way I could go was to qualify for, and earn, a bursary, which is not a scholarship. A scholarship is just basically a gift to pay for your education because of your outstanding performance. But the rest of us mere mortals basically would try to get bursaries which are based on economic need as well as academic performance and have strings attached. For instance, a company that needs electrical engineers may offer a few bursaries, which would pay for university education if you were granted one.

In exchange, you had to work for the company for a few years following graduation. Anglo-American awarded me a bursary, but I was committed to work on their mines during vacations and after graduation. Essentially, I was destined to become a section engineer, as they are called. It did not work out like that in the end, though, but we will revisit that later. At this stage, however, Anglo-American was paying for my education and boarding.

Wits was roughly an hour's drive from the racecourse. Although the university did not have a fraternity system like here in the States, I ended up living on campus, where there were halls of residence – two for men and two for women.

I lived in one of those residences, and it was a very different experience to someone going to boarding school in high school. With its rigorous rules and regulations, boarding school is almost like being in the army. University life, on the other hand, was very different from that highly structured setting; you were treated like an adult and had almost no rules.

Without anyone to guide you, you had to figure out how to handle the change, adjust to your new surroundings, and enter adulthood. A noteworthy feature of living in a residence (Res, as we called it) was the dining facilities, which served meals to the residents. Although it was institutional food, it wasn't as bad as being in prison and I think it was probably better than most high school boarding schools too. But it was still institutional food and it was very carb-centric, with everything cooked in vegetable oil, very low fat, margarine instead of butter. It was pretty much the same thing we ate at home, just less tasty. I always looked forward to the odd weekend when we could go home and actually enjoy Mom's cooking for a couple of days. I was 18 when I first showed up at Res and one of the first things I did once I had my own fridge in my room was to go out and buy some whole milk again.

Even though the Res food wasn't brilliant, I go back again to feeling really, really proud to be a part of the Res culture. So there were interfaculty leagues, made up of the different residences and university faculties in many sports like rugby, for instance. So the engineering group would have a team, the mining group would have a team, the dental students would have a team, and the medical students would have a team. Each of the different residences would have a team as well. And whenever the team was playing rugby, pretty much everybody went to support them without it being compulsory in any way. It was like my early high school days back in Rhodesia with war cries and a lot of noise – it was just an amazing atmosphere, and it was so awesome to be a part of that.

I played a lot of sports, but mostly contact sports and short sprint-type sports like rugby and squash, not endurance sports like running. I played rugby and represented our Res against other teams in the interfaculty league. They also had squash courts at our Res, and that's a very intense game. You can get really, really fit playing squash.

There was a Joburg marathon every year, and there was a group of guys in Res who got together to train to enter and run that marathon. I remember thinking once that this might be quite a bit of fun, so I thought I'd go and try it. I went out with this group of guys, and I found out later that they were all actually really good athletes. I started running with them and got pretty much two blocks down the road and I had to slow down and stop. In the end, I just walked back because I felt like I was dying. I thought, *I'm just not a marathon runner. I'm a rugby player and a squash player, but I can't do this marathon running thing.* For the rest of my days at university, that was how I thought of myself. But you will see later that when I was eventually doing my military service, it became apparent to me that it was not really the case. I found out that if I slowed down a little bit, I could run for a very long time.

That eventually led to my marathon running days in the years following my time in the army. Looking back, there's a saying that resonates with me now: 'You can't out-exercise a bad diet.' I was really fit, but under the hood, things were going awry, I just didn't know it yet.

At that stage, I didn't see myself as metabolically dysfunctional or ill, but it was creeping up on me. When I got older, that became a dysfunction that I felt like I needed to address. Eventually, I would decide to change how I ate by adopting a ketogenic diet, and everything would change for me.

CHAPTER 4

THE ARMY

At that time in South Africa, there was a compulsory two-year national service requirement for all males. Most young males went straight after high school, but if you got accepted into a university or college to continue with tertiary education, then you were able to get your service commitment postponed until you had finished that.

By the time I left university, I had deferred it as long as I could and it was time to go! I had to report for service by the next month, which was January. Because I did electrical engineering, I was assigned to the Signal Corp at Heidelberg, which was about an hour away from Joburg. (There it is again, it seems like everything's an hour's drive from Joburg?)

I ended up doing my three months of basic training and then got accepted into officer's training, which was another six or eight months, which was pretty much the rest of that year. By the second year, I was an officer. I think the real difference between training and being an officer was the food. During basic training, the food was pretty awful. But then, once I became an officer, I was able to eat in the officers' mess, where staff actually served you your food on a plate!

It was still a lot of rubbish – very low-fat everything, vegetable oils, margarine instead of butter – but at least it was relatively tasty. The chefs were experienced at making bad food taste palatable.

Sport was a big thing and the military was very keen to be represented wherever possible. The Heidelberg Gymnasium had a couple of rugby teams and hockey teams and if you played on a unit team in one of these sports, and participated in a match on the weekend, then you got a weekend pass.

In the beginning, I was playing rugby because that was what I played at school and at university. But we were playing in a very minor league since I wasn't really good enough to play in the first team (if you weren't an officer, then you had to be a provincial-level player to make it into the first team). I was still training and was not an officer at that stage, so I was relegated to the minor leagues, which was not fun at all.

It was basically just a bunch of thugs who just wanted to take their week's frustrations out on us, especially because we were, or at least a lot of us were English and there was always this undercurrent of friction between the 'Souties' (English people) and the Afrikaners. Sometimes it didn't seem to matter that there was a ball on the field at all, and since I was small compared to everybody else, I just got crushed. *But I'm getting out on pass, right?* Except I really just spent the weekend trying to recover from the beating I had received on the rugby field.

At that point, I remembered back when I was at university, I was thinking that I kind of felt like I wasn't a distance runner, but I started to realise, once I was in the army, that this wasn't the case. During training, we were split up into four sections, and they used to have these class competitions (why they didn't call them section competitions, I don't know). Each section would get allocated a couple of telephone poles and a couple of these big concrete paving stones, which they called 'marbles'. Then we had to run in our boots with our rifle and webbing, while sharing the load of the poles and marbles amongst the others in the section. The route was an off-road 21km course, which is basically a half-marathon.

One point that they drive into your brain incessantly in the military is that you don't leave anybody behind – everybody in the section has to finish together. So in order to help the less athletic guys in our section, I was often carrying an extra rifle. A couple of times, we even had someone draped over the telephone poles that we were carrying just because they couldn't continue anymore and we didn't want to slow down more than we had to, it was a race after all. Instead of waiting for them to recover, we draped them over the poles and carried them.

I would get back and think, *Wow, I just did a half marathon distance in boots and steel helmet with a rifle and all of this stuff! What if I just had a pair of running shoes and shorts on? I reckon I could easily run a half marathon race.*

While I was getting beaten up on the rugby field each weekend, there was a group of runners who were getting out on pass to run road races in defence colours. Pretoria is just north of Joburg and there are a ton of running clubs in those two cities. Each of them would put on a race once a year. Pretoria clubs had races on Saturdays and the Joburg clubs on Sundays so they were able to find a 10k, 15k or half marathon race somewhere within driving distance every weekend.

So I decided to apply to join this running group and quit the rugby team. The instructors would let them out on Friday night, they would run the race early Saturday or Sunday morning and they had the rest of the weekend off and would have to report back to camp around six o'clock on Sunday evening.

The instructors allowed me in, but I was literally the very last person to be allowed to join the group because more and more people had been starting to catch on and the officers decided that there were too many people taking advantage of this 'loophole' we had found. While they didn't mind the people who were genuine runners going out and doing this, they didn't want people doing it just to get out on pass. So they stopped it after me and I was really lucky because it had a huge impact on my life.

A couple of months later, I found out about a guy in South Africa named Professor Tim Noakes, who's now an absolute icon in the low-carb/ketogenic world. He wrote a book called *The Lore of Running* and it was pretty much considered the 'bible' for distance runners. A lot of it was focused towards what you needed to do in order to train for, and participate in, the Comrades Marathon, which is like a cult in South Africa.

It wasn't a matter of whether you were going to watch it on TV or not, it was a matter of where you were going to watch it. It was on TV the whole day. It is a 90 km race, roughly, which is about 55 miles over a very mountainous course. The cutoff time in those days was 11 hours (it's 12 now), but the TV coverage was 12 hours to cover the start and the dramatic final cut-off at 11 hours. When the gun fires after 11 hours, the organisers pull a fence across the finish and people who miss the cutoff, even by 1 second, are not even allowed to pass under the finish banner. Imagine that, after 11 hours on the road!

We used to get up early in the morning and watch it from start to finish. The people who lived relatively close to the course would actually all drive there, park the car, have a braai (barbeque) and spend the entire day sitting along the roadside at various points along the route. A lot of Prof's book was talking about preparing to do that race.

He also had this huge section on nutrition, and he was the one who initially introduced the dogma, I believe, that you really, really need carbohydrates to function as a distance runner. According to him, back then, we should be eating carbs all the time and then increase that intake substantially in the three or four days before the race (he called it 'carb loading'). We'll learn later how he did a 180 on this idea.

I remember we were doing one of our field exercises and we dug these little foxholes and put a tarpaulin over them to protect us from the rain and weather. It was really miserable. But we had some down-time now and again. I remember having a little lantern in there and actually reading this book, and that was when I was inspired to attempt the Comrades Marathon at some time, which I did a bit further down the road.

CHAPTER 5

ADULT LIFE

As I mentioned earlier, I had acquired a bursary from Anglo-American, and there was a commitment for me to work on the mines for two years once I'd finished university and my army training. A lot of bursaries actually required four years, so two years was actually minimal, but still, I was going to have to work underground on a gold mine – the deepest gold mine in South Africa is 4km or 2.5 miles – for at least two years.

I had been assigned to a gold mine that was, funnily enough, an hour's drive or so from Joburg in a town called Klerksdorp. I had a few weeks between when I finished with the army and when I was due to start on the mines in January, so I started hanging out with this friend of mine who was doing triathlons. I started canoeing and cycling and we were doing these little triathlons.

The weekend before I was due to report for work at the mine in Klerksdorp, there was this triathlon there, in the same town. It was canoeing, cycling and running and we went there and participated. Afterwards, as we drove back home to Joburg, we were on an open road, pretty much in the middle of nowhere and I was in the passenger seat. We had our paddles between the driver's seat and the passenger seat, and our bikes and boats strapped to the roof rack on the top of the car. Halfway along this straight open road with nothing on it, there was a garage on the side of the road. We decided that we wanted to pull off and get something to drink.

I've been told this because I literally don't remember, but I believe I was leaning down in my footwell, trying to get my wallet out of my bag, as my friend turned across the traffic without seeing an oncoming car and we got t-boned. The car literally hit us at my door and I was in a really bad way.

Just a quick segue here: while I was in hospital, my dad came into town and, as an ex-police officer, he did a very thorough investigation himself. From what he could find out, there was an undercover, or off-duty, cop who pulled onto the road in the opposite direction to us at great speed which is why Ian didn't see him coming. He was the one who hit us and then he just drove away. Although I doubt his car was driveable so maybe he called a friend to fetch him, but the bottom line is, he fled the scene. Dad still has all his notes in tiny writing in a little notebook to this day. He took all this to the local cops, but nothing ever came of it.

———

I often say that, when I heard more and more about what state I was in, I really don't know why or how I didn't die that day. I like to believe it's because I still had work to do in starting these organisations that I'm now running and being part of and helping so many people. The theory is that I hit the back of my head on the little attachment where the seat belt comes out of the door frame. Then, since we got hit in my door, I was crushed between the caved-in door and the paddles, and I suffered a compression fracture of my collarbone. I also had three ribs that were dislocated from the sternum and a vertebra in my spine that was dislodged. Chiropractic adjustments helped later on but almost 40 years later, if you run your finger down my sternum, you can still feel where the ribs are dislocated. Run your finger down my spine and you can feel the vertebra that is out of place. But that was nothing compared to the head injury.

Apparently, I was just sort of semi-conscious, rocking backwards and forwards, just moaning. There was another friend of ours who had come to do the race as well, and he left to go home a little later than us. He said that when he came upon the crash, the only reason he realised it was us was because of our bikes and canoes. The whole roof rack had come off in one piece and it kind of floated off to the side and was literally sitting on the side of the road with two bikes and two canoes still attached. So this mate of mine was trying to get past the accident, recognised the bikes and the canoes, and he knew it was our stuff.

So he stopped and came and had a look. He said that's when he noticed I was just sitting in the passenger seat, rocking backwards and forwards. We were taken to the local Klerksdorp hospital, where I suppose they did the best they could, but it wasn't the greatest. I had this massive brain injury that they weren't equipped to deal with.

So apparently, after a week or two, they transferred me to a facility in Joburg that was basically a neurological centre. That was what this facility focused on. In the meantime, I literally couldn't feel anything, at least that is what I was told, because I don't remember. I was told that at one stage while I was still in the Klerksprop hospital, my family had come and were visiting and they wanted to do a lumbar puncture, which I was told is really painful. I was lying on my side and bracing for the pain. I was a bit grumpy, saying, 'Guys, come on. How long am I going to have to lie like this?'

And the nurse said, 'No, we're finished.'

I literally didn't even feel the pressure from them trying to stick this needle into my back. I didn't feel a thing.

That was the other problem with the collarbone break. If you look at the progression of x-rays, in the first one you can see this crack through the collarbone. But over time, they took these progressive x-rays. I wouldn't keep my arm still, because I couldn't feel any pain. Eventually, this crack became disjointed, and the bones came apart and were offset from each other but still touching. Then, after a bit more time, about a half-inch gap developed between the two different pieces of the collarbone. They would strap me into this straitjacket kind of thing, but because the collarbone was broken, it was almost like I could dislocate my shoulder.

So I would just manipulate my shoulder forward, like Houdini, and pull my arm out of this restraint again. The doctors, my mom, everybody, were just going absolutely crazy, but I couldn't feel anything. So I kept doing it.

By now, the orthopaedic surgeon needed to plate my collarbone, but the neurosurgeon wouldn't allow him to give me an anaesthetic to operate because I had this massive swelling on my brain.

I couldn't see anything either. I couldn't focus. Only if I closed one eye could I see out of the other eye. But when I looked with both eyes, it was just a big blur because the two eyes couldn't focus on the same point.

Later, people told me that they even hated talking to me during that time because it was like talking to a chameleon where my two eyes would move independently of each other. I actually thought that that was a lot of rubbish, but I've heard since that it's a real thing, it actually does happen.

Finally, I got to go home, but I was obviously pretty much house-bound and I was pretty bummed that I hadn't been able to do any exercise. So I found a gym that was just about a mile walk or so up the road from where I was staying. I was wearing this patch on my one eye so that I could see with the other eye. I would walk up to the gym and go and get on the exercise bike there. I still had my arm in a sling, but I was now at least cognisant enough of the fact that I really needed to try and keep the arm still in order to not do any more damage before it could get plated.

So there I was in the gym with a sling on my arm and a patch on my eye, and I would work really hard on the exercise bike. I actually got a decent amount of exercise in that way, which helped me a bit mentally, I think, as well. But it used to take me a long time to walk up there because on the way there I had to cross this double-lane road where there were two lanes going each way with this little island in the middle.

I remember one day looking up the road and seeing this car that I thought was a long way away, so I stepped into the road to cross it. Suddenly, there was screeching of tyres and smoke everywhere. Due to the lack of depth perception while wearing the eye patch, I couldn't gauge the distance of the cars. I very nearly died, *again*, stepping out like that right in front of a car that I thought was far away.

After that, I didn't trust myself anymore. So I would look one way and literally only cross to the island when I could see no cars at all. Then I'd look the other way and do the same thing before crossing the road completely. And that was my life, literally going up to the gym pretty much every day that I could and doing some exercise and coming back.

Reading wasn't an option. Even watching TV wasn't easy because I really couldn't see. I suppose I watched some with just one eye, but I don't remember that detail clearly.

Eventually, it got to the point where the swelling had gone down in my brain enough that the neurosurgeon was prepared to give permission for the orthopaedic surgeon to go in and plate the collarbone. So they went in and did that, but I still couldn't see properly.

Finally, I remember waking up one day and opening my eyes and actually seeing the ceiling. It didn't even register immediately that, *Hey, I can see the ceiling.* Literally 30 seconds later, it all went fuzzy again.

Then I realised that for a moment there, I had actually actually been able to see the ceiling. Over the next few days, that 30 seconds would get longer and longer. I would wake up and I could see for a bit. And then it would revert again. Finally, after a couple of weeks, I was able to see through the whole day.

Before this happened I was starting to think about work again. I really didn't want to go and work on the mines if I could help it. I'd done some vacation work there, and I'd had a glimpse of what my job would be and what my life would be after regaining my eyesight. I really didn't want to do that. So I had managed to find a software company in Joburg, literally 20 minutes drive from where I lived, that was prepared to buy me out, to pay off my bursary from the mines and have me come and work for them, assuming my eyesight came right.

Once I was able to see again, I contacted them and said, 'Hey, I'm ready to start working.' I still had to get a lift into work and have someone to pick me up again afterwards, because I didn't trust myself and I didn't know whether halfway down the freeway my vision would suddenly go again. So it was a couple of weeks where I was insistent that I get a lift before I eventually realised, *OK, I'm getting through the day and my vision is not going to fail me again.*

I started driving myself. It was probably four months after the accident that I actually drove again for the first time. Now that the collarbone was plated – I think even before they took the stitches out – I'd gone out on the road and started running again.

I think one of the things I was really, really concerned about was that I knew I had a head injury and my vision was affected but I wasn't sure if my limbs were going to function properly again. I had at least been able to ride the bike, so it couldn't have been that bad, although that was a stationary bike and I didn't know how my balance would be on a real bike. As it turns out, my balance has never really been 100% again. I noticed that the most when I eventually got back in the canoe but I've kind of adapted, I guess.

I still didn't know what running was going to be like, so I got out as soon as I could and started running and I was actually fine, I think, because I'd been able to maintain a reasonable amount of fitness on the exercise bike. I went for a couple of miles – I don't know, maybe even a 5k or 8k run – and I was fine.

So my vision was improving, and I was adapting where needed. My balance was slightly affected, but I was adapting there too. However, the biggest issue for me was – and still is – that my short-term memory was shot to pieces. I could remember things in my past, but I would forget what I was saying really easily. I was really struggling to find the words, even the easy words that obviously were in my vocabulary and were right there on the tip of my tongue. While I was speaking I knew what I wanted to say, but I often couldn't retrieve – and still can't often retrieve – words that I needed. I frequently have to resort to explaining what the meaning of the word is that I am trying to find, much like verbal charades.

Back when I was just getting back on the road, I had no idea where this path of recovery would lead and where I would end up and it was quite an anxious time. Being able to go out and run and sort of clear my mind and forget about it; I think that was very powerful. It helped me recover mentally from this whole ordeal, much more so than anything else. While I was out running I was starting to dream about this day when I would go and run that 55-mile race, the Comrades Marathon. So yeah, running helped.

While I'm talking about the brain injury, I wish I knew then what I know now. I came to realise that once you eliminate carbohydrates, sugar, processed foods and all this junk from your diet, it actually has amazing effects on brain injuries – neurological conditions and mental health as well. We'll learn all about that as we go further.

At this point of the story, I've started to go to work, and that's a whole new phase in my life. This new company I joined was a software company. I trained as an electrical engineer, software engineering didn't exist when I was studying and was literally a new discipline. When I was at university, we maybe did two or three courses on computer programming. But now software engineering has grown into a whole new engineering discipline – so software engineers were in high demand. I basically became a software engineer and went through a couple of different jobs. Eventually I ended up at a company that did satellite TV.

These two guys had come up with the idea of developing a digital satellite TV system. And they had tried to sell it in America, but the Americans had so much money invested in the analogue systems back then. They were actually the first ones to come up with satellite

TV, but it was an analogue system, long before digital came along – those huge dishes we used to see out in the garden. They just couldn't get their heads around the fact that digital was going to be so much better than what they had. The new digital dishes were tiny, and you could just bolt them onto the roof of your house. You could get 10, 15 channels sometimes onto one satellite transponder, instead of just one with the old system. So it was much cheaper. Eventually, everything was going to go digital, but the Americans couldn't see it at that time.

So these guys came home and found a local bank to bankroll them to start developing these boxes. But there was a terrorist situation going on by now and a lot of international pressure to establish a black government. – it was before Nelson Mandela had been released. There were sanctions imposed on South Africa so it was very difficult to get hold of electronic parts and components for them to build these boxes that they had designed.

They structured the company by basing half of it in Holland, and half of it in South Africa. Basically the head end side, the transmission side of the system, was all designed and developed in Holland. The receiver side, the set-top box that sat on top of your TV back in the days when you could still sit a box on top of a TV; all that development was done in South Africa.

That was the team that I was a part of. The company was registered in Holland, that was how they were able to get around the sanctions and still be able to source parts and whatever they needed to build these boxes. I ended up spending a lot of time in Holland. We were building the box for the European market at the time, so the satellite footprint is there in Europe.

In South Africa, we couldn't see the satellite. We had these test systems that mimicked the satellite feed that we could use to test the box that we were developing but when we actually sent the box over to Europe at the end of the day, and they connected it to a real satellite feed, what worked on the test system didn't work at all.

Obviously, there was a lot of finger-pointing going on. The head-end guys are saying that it's a receiver problem, and the receiver guys are saying it's the transmission side. The only way to really solve that is to put both sides in the same room, under the satellite footprint, and solve the problem, so that happened a lot. That's why I ended up spending a lot of time in Holland. And I really hated it. For me, I mean, coming from an area where there were lots of mountains and sunshine, I was running through the hills and the mountains all the time and now the environment is totally flat. In South Africa, we have sunshine all the time. And whenever I was in Holland, it was grey and miserable and raining.

I felt like the sky was right on my head. I don't know if it was particular to the company that I was working for but I found the people very unfriendly and grey as well. When any of us went over there from South Africa, we stayed in a hotel across the road from the office. In all the time we spent there, which was a lot, no one ever invited us to even come to dinner with them. No one invited us to their houses over the weekend, when we were there over the weekend. I often tell the story that, if it were the other way around – if we had people coming and sitting in our offices because they were developing something for our South African or African market – it would have been a different story.

When guys came from overseas, we would literally fight over who was going to have them back to our house to come and watch rugby or cricket or just come and have dinner or whatever. It was like this rush as the guys came in the door; they got pounced on, everyone was saying, 'You guys, you need to come to our house for the weekend.'

It wasn't really quite as insane as that, but it kind of seemed like that sometimes. It was just a different culture in Holland and I was not enjoying my time there.

Anyway, I was adapting to work as an engineer. There were times when I would be working on designs and would have to present them to get feedback from everybody else. Then you incorporate that feedback into your design and start coding it, but having to do a little presentation like that used to scare me to death. First, I was so fearful of forgetting what I was saying and going blank or, second, I would remember what I wanted to say but couldn't find the words. So that was an enormous stress on me. Down the road, when I became more senior, I became a leader on these projects. I always used to get the junior guys to do the presentations, even if it was something I really should have been doing myself. If there was any way that I wouldn't have to stand up in front of people and have to deal with that fear and that stress, I would find it.

CHAPTER 6

MOVING TO THE U.S.

C hanges were happening in South Africa; Nelson Mandela was released, sanctions were a thing of the past, and the new South Africa was 'flavour of the month'. We thought that they were going to relocate everybody to South Africa at that point.

We thought they were going to combine and merge everything and everybody would end up working in Joburg. But then, just out of the blue, we got notified that they had decided to do quite the opposite. To this day, I have no idea why, but they relocated the set-top box component of the business to Hoofddorp in Holland, where the head-end transmission side was being developed. As employees, we were offered amazing packages to move to Holland, but as I mentioned earlier, I really didn't enjoy being there. I found the people pretty difficult – although, again, that could just have been the company I was at – so the thought of moving there and that place becoming my home didn't really appeal to me at all. It just wasn't for me.

No other companies in South Africa produced digital satellite TV set-top boxes, which was what our engineering experience was.

We just didn't know what was coming next. There wasn't an opportunity for us to find another job unless we were going to start again and learn to write software for some other device. We would have to learn a different job because our niche expertise was in the set-top boxes now and writing software for them.

A few of us decided to at least look elsewhere instead of going to Holland. We thought maybe there's some other country in the world that we could go to where we could find a job. The US had just got to that point where they realised that it didn't matter how much money they had invested in all the analogue satellite TV systems – the world was changing, and everything was going digital. So they started to embrace that idea and began to try to build these digital systems themselves so engineers who were capable in that field were in high demand. There was a friend of ours, Ivan McLean, who had moved to the US about a year earlier and was working for a company called Radyne in San Diego so another friend, Glenn Forrester, and I travelled to America. There was a job fair in the San Francisco Bay Area, so we stayed with Glenn's cousin who lived there and attended it. We literally had four or five interviews each come out of that show.

Glenn had another cousin who lived in San Diego, so we went there next. We didn't find anybody in San Diego who was at the fair, but we somehow managed to organise a couple of interviews at companies in the area, one of which was Radyne, which Ivan organised. I remember it was at the peak of the dot-com boom when this was going on. The traffic in the San Francisco Bay area was just insane, especially for all of us coming from South Africa, where we were only used to a two-lane highway. Now, we are sometimes in six and seven lanes that were at a standstill for hours on end on each side of the freeway. Rush hour in the morning and evening was something to behold and I couldn't cope with it. We actually borrowed his cousin's car and drove down to San Diego. I remember a couple of things about driving there. First, we had to drive through Los Angeles on the way down, which was just as bad as the Bay Area, but it was as we started to clear the outskirts of LA and head towards San

Diego that we really detected this difference in attitude on the road. It was the most amazing thing; the aggression and road rage that we experienced driving in San Francisco and then down through LA was crazy. But then as we drove south and neared San Diego, it kind of evaporated. I remember thinking to myself, *If I get offered a job here, I'm coming because I just don't think I can cope with the traffic in the Bay Area.*

It turns out that the traffic in San Diego wasn't that much better, to be honest, but the difference in the vibe during rush hour in the morning and evening was clear. We were on the road, and we literally sensed the difference. My buddy Glenn experienced the same thing. We ended up getting offers from a bunch of different companies, including Radyne, and we decided to take that offer and join Ivan at Radyne. There was one other guy who decided to move to the States as well, but he didn't come with us to that job fair. I think he contacted Ivan in San Diego, who organised an interview for him. He literally flew out specifically for that interview and he got an offer too, and so there were four of us altogether at Radyne. We started working and it was a big thing to come from – I don't want to say a backward country, but South Africa compared to the States was very different – it was just like everything was on a much bigger scale in the US.

I think my first real shock was going out to dinner and finding out you could order a starter that came on this massive plate and was bigger than anything I'd ever seen as a main course in Europe or in South Africa. The main course was still to follow. Then the local people would suggest to you that you just need to get a 'doggy bag', a box for your leftovers that you can take home and eat later. Now when I look back on it and I visualise what was on the plate, I remember that it was so full of carbs you couldn't believe it. And it's not just the carbs, it's the amount of food on the plate as well. I was always taught to finish what was on my plate. That was my mom's big thing, so I would get this giant plate of food, and I was trying to force myself to finish it. It's not just all the carbs but just a huge excess of food – nobody should be eating that much.

I would say that we didn't find the people nearly as friendly in San Diego as we were used to in South Africa. But it was better than Holland. We weren't part of their cliques, so we didn't get invited home with them for a very long time. The four of us just used to hang out together on weekends. That was our social group, so I suppose we had a little clique of our own. I sometimes think maybe if we hadn't had that group and it was just me or any one of them alone, maybe we would have infiltrated these other groups or cliques more quickly and easily because we wouldn't have had anybody else to socialise with.

I think our natural way of socialising was to have a 'braai' (barbeque), as we called it in South Africa. What I should have done on the weekends was go get a bunch of meat, arrange a place where I could cook it outside on a fire, and invite some folks around. I don't think anyone would have refused. If they had come over, we could have had more casual conversations than we managed at work. Perhaps we would have made friends in the States much faster as a result.

We had been brought into Radyne to build set-top boxes for a company called Matsushita in Japan. There was a lot of political turmoil within that organisation. We were doing a really good job and were way ahead of schedule with the development, yet suddenly, the project was just pulled out from under us and cancelled. It was the only set-top box project that Radyne had and they were really struggling to find a place for us now, so we started looking around at other companies to see where we could move to. It was really quite fortuitous that the building next door to us was Motorola.

I wasn't even in the country at the time – I think I was in South Africa working on some set-top box thing; I forget what it was – and the rest of the team got an interview with Motorola to go and move over there and work with them. Our team had a Vietnamese guy named Hoa, who was just the most incredible engineer we'd ever come across. He was brilliant. We also had this American colleague named Ron on our team, who was like our technical guru, so when we needed to get special probes in there for testing and trying to develop software, he would be the one who would get these boxes and open them up and do all of the soldering. If one of our boxes stopped working, he was the one who would troubleshoot it. We got on so well with him, too.

As I said, I wasn't even there, but the other guys went across to Motorola, and because digital set-top box engineers were so hard to find in those days, they literally laid down the law and insisted that the whole team come across. I mean, I actually didn't even have an interview at Motorola. The other guys interviewed, and they insisted Hoa, Ron, and I come too. All six of us got new jobs at Motorola, so they referred to us as the six-pack – sometimes not in a very warm way. Anyway, we were the six-pack and that was where I started to get into a more management-type position. Until then, I'd just been another engineer working on the software on these boxes. However, working at Motorola, I eventually became the project manager for one of the projects we were working on. Eventually, that was what got me into the international work that I was able to do.

I was back running again. Back in South Africa, I had developed really bad Achilles tendonitis from wearing the wrong shoes while training for Comrades – literally to the extent where I could feel big ridges of scar tissue on my Achilles tendons if I ran my fingers up and down. It was constantly really painful, but I used to run through the pain, and after a while, the endorphins would kick in, and the pain would subside. Obviously, I was constantly making this injury worse, and eventually, I just couldn't do it anymore. I went to a very famous orthopaedic surgeon who did an operation on me called an 'Achilles release'. Basically, he goes in and removes the entire sheath of the Achilles tendon, which now has all this scar tissue attached to it. Then he literally slits the tendon vertically so that it increases blood flow and supports proper healing.

That put me out for a few years. Before that, I ran Comrades four times. I hadn't run for a couple of years, but after recovering from that injury, I ran my fifth one literally two weeks before I moved to the US. The big thing with that race is that if you run ten of them, then they retire your number, and they basically present you with this big green piece of material with a laurel wreath and your number embroidered on it for you to frame and you get to keep that number and no one ever gets to run in it again. It's really a big deal. If you ever run again after that, your number (bib) is actually green. Everybody on the road knows what it means and they are so supportive. You get a lot of extra cheering if you are running in your green number. I had never really thought about trying to attain mine, especially after I'd moved to the States. I never intended to go back and run it again, but then I got into running here, and I ended up running a couple of different marathons. One of them was on Catalina Island. It is a very mountainous, tough race, and a couple of local friends of mine that I used to run with came and did that one with me.

The next day, we were sitting and having lunch on the waterfront of this beautiful island and as we were eating, I started telling them about Comrades.

By the time we left that island, everyone had decided we were going to go to South Africa and run Comrades. I think it was the following year that the three of us went back and ran, and that was now my sixth one. It was weird. It was like the tipping point. Suddenly I was on the other side of that tipping point, and I was closer to ten than I'd ever been. It was a thing now, and I felt I needed to keep going back so that I could earn my green number. Over the years, I did that, but if I look back now, I see that my knees were really taking a lot of strain. My Achilles tendons were fine. I'd had that operation and changed my shoes and I never had problems with my Achilles tendons again, but just the stress and the inflammation that was building up from all those 100-mile weeks was starting to take their toll. I got my green number but it was really hard, so after I did ten, I really didn't want to go and do it again, even though that meant I would never run in my green number.

I actually did start a campaign once to go back and run just once in green. I met a girl who was working on both Pam and me as a physiotherapist, and I persuaded her to come back and run it with me. I helped train her with the idea that we would both run it and I would get the chance to run in my green number. Then I twisted my ankle really badly at one point during training and I wasn't able to continue training. We went back, but I didn't run it. She did, though, and it was an epic experience for her. It's impossible to describe what it feels like to cross that finish line. So I've never actually ran in my green number, but I still think it's quite an achievement to have earned it. I think that the most important part is just setting your mind to something and becoming so disciplined that, no matter what, you get out there and you do the training.

I spent many hours on the road out there alone. Some people are ok with their own company, but for me, after a while it sometimes gets a bit old. But I kept doing it because I had this goal in mind, which helped me in later life. When something presents itself that I need to do or that I decide I need to get done, it's kind of hard to stop me until I get it done. I think the experience of trying to run the Comrades so many times really helped with that. I don't know, maybe it made me better at getting the job done.

One of the big things I mentioned earlier was that I had read Professor Tim Noakes' book *The Lore of Running* while I was still in the army. That book inspired me to run Comrades for the first time and one of the things I remember is that he's got this whole chapter on teaching how important carbohydrates are for running and especially carb loading a few days before the race. It was something that occurred to me later on when I saw the changes that happened when I began to eliminate carbohydrates and sugar from my life.

During the carb-loading phase, I forced all these carbs down for three or four days before these races that I'd run. Yet every single time I was standing on the start line, I used to feel like I was literally going to struggle to run to the corner. I just felt shocking. I was so fit, standing there each time with so much expectation of how well I could do and yet feeling like I wanted to die. I always used to think that it was nerves because everything in my whole life was about training for Comrades. Everything I did was focused on what I should be doing and what was best for me to be able to perform on the day of Comrades. Suddenly, every time I'm standing on the start line thinking, *How the hell am I going to get up this mountain for 55 miles when I feel like I can't even get to the corner?*

It was only much later when everything changed for me that I looked back and realised that it wasn't nerves, it was just that I'd poisoned myself with carbohydrates.

CHAPTER 7

A WHOLE NEW WORLD

At this point, I'm in the States, I'm getting older, I've run my 10th Comrades Marathon, and I'm still running.

We always went to Catalina Island for their marathon, which was a big thing. I didn't run a ton of marathons anymore. I always used to just run most of them for training. But Catalina was an exception. A few of us used to go out there together, and it was almost like a camping trip. The run was just a small part of the whole weekend. It was an amazing weekend on the island.

But as I mentioned earlier, my knees were getting really sore, and I was putting on just a little bit of weight each year. And I used to think that I was lazy because I wasn't running a hundred miles a week. I thought that putting on a little weight all the time was why I couldn't run anymore. But my muscles were sore, my knees were sore, and running just really wasn't fun anymore.

I was doing it because I thought I needed to keep doing it to stay healthy. But yeah, it just wasn't fun anymore and I felt like I was actually hating life because it was so painful and so miserable to go out and run every day.

That kind of influenced everything else. So instead of running being this thing that was making my life better, it had started making it worse. But I continued to do it because I thought if I didn't, I was just being lazy.

During that time, Pam and I started to do martial arts. There's a mixed martial arts crowd that we got introduced to that was just a really fun crowd. So we started to do that, but it was a really long drive. It was about a 40-minute drive from where we used to stay downtown to this gym where they would train. Originally, we were doing four workouts – four classes a week. That was four days a week of driving all the way up there and all the way back in the evening. After a while, we decided, 'Okay, let's just do two classes instead.' So the class we went to was always the last class of the day, the seniors class.

But the juniors class was full of teenagers who were around the age of 18. They were big kids. Our coach basically said that we were welcome to come and do that class as well. So we did that class and literally had a five-minute break and then did the next class. So we were doing 90 minutes of intense martial arts workouts twice a week.

I felt tired when we got home at night, but the next day I was so stiff that I literally felt like I had to crawl to the bathroom; it was that bad. I intended to go for a run every day, but on these days, I would think, *No. I can't go out and run like this.* It was ridiculous.

I was running less, but I was attending the martial arts workouts, which were very intense. So I thought, *Okay, I'm getting enough exercise there.* It didn't really faze me that I wasn't running as much. I was hating running anyway. So it wasn't that difficult to back off there a little bit. But, I just felt like something was wrong, I just didn't know what.

We actually got involved with a bunch of different businesses because, at that time I had been trying to get out of the engineering field to try to do something on my own. I tried a bunch of different things, but nothing stuck. I was a perfectionist, always trying to make sure that everything was perfect before I launched it. When it turned out that it wasn't what other people wanted, and I didn't have the money or the strength anymore to try to fix it. Each one was a really big fail.

At that point, I met this very influential guy at one of the businesses that I got involved with. He actually served on Marine One, which is the helicopter that flies the president around. You don't get to do that by being just an average guy, so he was pretty impressive.

He had become involved in a startup company that was trying to sell exogenous ketones. At that time, I didn't know what a ketone was, but I got an email from him in July of 2015 that was titled something like *Ketones: A Better Source of Fuel than Glucose*. And it was just the right time for me. I believe everything in this world comes down to timing. And it was time. My knees were sore. I hated running. I was miserable. I knew something was wrong, but I didn't know what. And because I was a runner, I obviously thought of glucose as the best source of fuel. That was what we all totally believed in.

If this had happened at any other time in my life, I would have just blown it off completely. But the day that I got that email, my ears pricked up. I started to look into it. For the next three weeks, I studied everything that I could find about the ketogenic diet and ketosis and what that all meant. I literally buried myself in it. And by the end of those three weeks, it explained everything.

It explained what I mentioned a little bit back about feeling like I was going to die on the starting line of the Comrades Marathon back when I was in my early thirties and running those ultra-long races. I had all these problems that I was experiencing now as I got older and was putting on this little bit of weight and feeling sore all the time. I understand why now, but at the time, I didn't know anything about the physiology and metabolism involved in consuming excessive carbohydrates, which led to the problems that I was experiencing.

When I started looking at it as a scientist, it just explained everything. The startup ketone company had run out of product, and I wasn't able to order any of them. So I thought, why take these ketones exogenously? Why not just do the diet and get the full benefits of the metabolic changes that happen when you eliminate carbohydrates? That is what I had learned about the whole process.

We decided to do it. I said to Pam, 'We're going shopping,' and she nearly fell off the chair.

And then I said, 'Hang on, I've got to get my list.' She said, 'Wait, what? You're going shopping, *and* you've got a list? Something's up here!'

At that point, I think I had kind of mentioned it to her, but I hadn't really told her in-depth about everything that I'd learned and why I felt like I wanted to do this. I just dragged her to the store. Basically, what you learn is that if you do this ketogenic diet and you're trying to eliminate carbohydrates and sugars and processed food, the main thing you have to do is avoid all the aisles in the supermarket!

Literally, the only things you want to eat are around the perimeter of the store. You mainly go to the meats, veggies, dairy, and eggs. I used to cut every little bit of fat off the meat that I ate. Now I'm buying a ribeye steak, which is about the fattiest cut around. We were buying heavy cream, full cream Greek yoghurt, and all of these items that I'd learned over the last few weeks that we needed to be eating in order to get into ketosis and live this ketogenic lifestyle.

We took it all home, and Pam kept saying to me, 'Where am I going to get my vitamins from if we're not going to eat, you know, bread and cereal?'

I told her, 'There are way more nutrients and vitamins that we require for our bodies, in spades, in the meat and all these ingredients that we were buying than you will ever find in fortified bread and cereal and all this processed food, where it's all been added in, if it's there at all, and completely bio-unavailable if it is, your body can't even use it.'

The very first thing that we ate as we adopted this lifestyle was the ribeye steaks that I bought. In the complex where we were staying, there were these braais outside. I went down and lit a fire on one, and we cooked these two ribeye steaks.

I put them on a plate and brought them inside. You could see all the fat on the steak and it was just dripping with rendered fat too. This is such a vivid memory for me. The fat that was rendering out of the steak was sloshing around on the bottom of the plate.

I started giggling, looked at Pam, and said, 'Are we really going to eat this?' But I had read enough of the science to really believe that this was what we were supposed to be doing. I was so programmed against fat that I basically had to gag down the first couple of bites I took of that steak because my mind was telling me that it was bad for me, or at least the fat was.

And, it was really hard for me to swallow. But then I had another piece and another piece and another piece. And after a while, I thought to myself, *You know what? This actually tastes really, really good.* I mean, I love meat. I'm from Africa, right? But this steak was like a whole different ball game. So that's where it started. That was the beginning of our journey down the rabbit hole!

Back then, there was very little information on the ketogenic diet, really. It was still considered very taboo. Now you can't look on the internet anywhere without seeing tons of information about it.

But that wasn't the case back then; we didn't know what we were doing. We did stuff wrong, we struggled with things, and we just bungled our way through it, I suppose. We eventually found out about a food-tracking app that we started to use, and that helped.

We didn't know it then, but we soon found out that so many things contain sugar, either naturally, or added, or both. For instance, somehow we thought that watermelons didn't have a lot of sugar in them, for some reason. I don't know why we thought that, but that right there was a big thing.

We used to go and buy a whole watermelon at the supermarket and we cleared a couple of shelves so that we could keep it at the bottom of the fridge. Then, each night after our dinner, I would cut this big slice of watermelon and cut it in half, and we'd each have half. That had a lot to do with why we saw our progress stall at one point. After learning this, we thought, *Oh, wait a minute, there's a ton of sugar in watermelon*. We stopped eating it, and suddenly, our weight loss started to happen again, and we were back on track.

My weight started to come down. But we kept having these stalls. We would work out what we were doing wrong, and then it would start coming down again. I didn't mention it at the beginning, but along with all these issues I was having back before we started, I also stood on the scale and discovered that I was 35 pounds over what I considered my normal weight. I was shocked.

So that was one of the other things that had happened a couple of days before I got this email. That became my biggest thing, to get this weight off so that I could start feeling better. I could hopefully take 35 pounds off, and my running would be better.

But what started to happen was that other issues started to clear up that I hadn't known about, or even considered. I had this huge inflammation in my knees that cleared up. The recovery time from any effort was incredible. Earlier, I was talking about those 90-minute martial arts sessions that we would do. Now, I would come home, and the next day, I would bounce out of bed and go for a run. It was astounding.

One of the most significant changes was how my brain was affected. I told you about the accident I had, the brain injury I experienced, and how it impacted me, particularly with short-term memory and trying to retrieve words. That didn't go away, but somehow I felt like it was happening less frequently. You know, previously, I would forget what I was saying all the time. But as I changed the way I ate, it started happening less frequently.

I still struggle to retrieve words sometimes, but it has improved, and I am enormously grateful for that. And remember how I suffered from anxiety having to give presentations, and I always tried to get out of it? I was open to it now, even though I would have never considered doing it before.

I learned a lot from psychiatrist Dr Georgia Ede. She talks about how changing the way you eat really helps with anxiety and other mental health conditions. I think that's how it helped me. Yes, I knew I might forget what I was saying on the stage or struggle to find words, but I wasn't anxious about it, and I wasn't afraid of it anymore.

When we first adopted this diet, we were really flying under the radar since it was so unconventional that we didn't tell anyone about it.

But after a few months, we noticed huge differences. In those days, my parents still lived in South Africa. So we would have a call with them once a week and just chat. It was almost a standing thing: Sunday morning our time was evening for them there, so it was good timing.

About three months into this journey, during one of these chats, we just had to fess up. I think my mom was the first person we really told about it. We started telling her about what this diet involved and how great we were feeling and she said to me, 'That sounds like the Tim Noakes' diet.' As you know by now, I was a big Tim Noakes fan, he was like my hero.

I said, 'No way!' I jumped on my laptop while we were still on the call and started searching for him.

A few years later, we ended up doing an interview with him for our YouTube channel and he told us that he had received an email that was pitched something like 'Lose Five Kilos (11lbs) in a couple of weeks without hunger', written by Jeff Volek and Stephen Phinney. Tim thought, *There's no way*, but he really respected Jeff and Steve. He went out and somehow he managed to get his hands on that book in South Africa.

He started reading it and it did the same thing for him as my research had done for me. It was like this big epiphany: *What? So much of what I've been teaching people my whole life, my whole career, is basically rubbish?* He told me in the interview that he was supposed to be going to do a lecture about marathon running in Sweden. Anyway, he was like me and had been gradually putting on a little bit of weight all the time. He felt almost self-conscious of the fact that he was going to be speaking to all these runners about marathon running when he was carrying this extra weight and didn't look, or feel, like a marathon runner anymore, and he wasn't running well either.

That was extra motivation for him to just try this. So he did, and the weight came off, and he looked fabulous, so he went off happily and did his lecture. At that time, he had developed diabetes as well, with an HbA1C of 6.5% (48 mmol/mol). A little while later, he found that his A1C had dropped to 5.5% (37 mmol/mol), which is no longer even in the prediabetes range.

He's supposed to be retired now, but after that, he says that he's committing the rest of his life to trying to correct the misinformation that he was a part of putting out there during his career. For a scientist and a doctor to put his hand up and say he was totally wrong and would try to make it right takes enormous courage.

I think everybody in this community has undying respect for Tim and the fact that he is prepared to stand up and admit that he had been wrong and that he wanted to put it right. He made a video of himself literally tearing the pages out of that book and saying that he was totally wrong and that he was sorry and he was busy writing a revision for the book.

Tim became very involved in trying to re-educate all of us in terms of what to eat just for general health, and especially for distance running and endurance events. He wants to teach us how we should actually be preparing for a race nutritionally, which is so different to what he had been teaching before.

So he became very well known online amongst the low-carb/ketogenic community, and he was very active on Twitter. At one point, somebody put out a tweet about weaning a baby, and Tim's response basically caused a global meltdown. The lady was doing an LCHF (Low-Carb High-Fat) diet, which is what the low-carb diet is often referred to and, in its strictest form, is the ketogenic diet. Her tweet said, '*Is LCHF eating ok for breastfeeding mums? Worried about all the dairy + cauliflower = wind for babies??*' (you'll learn more about LCHF later). Tim replied, '*Baby doesn't eat the dairy and cauliflower.*

Just very healthy high fat breast milk. Key is to ween [sic] baby onto LCHF.' and the world was knocked off its axis!

As described by Bill Gifford in his article 'The Silencing of Tim Noakes', a Johannesburg dietitian named Claire Strydom, who was then head of the Association for Dietetics in South Africa (ADSA), read this and was horrified that Noakes would recommend such a radical diet for an infant. She reported him to the Health Professions Council of SA (HPCSA), and a few months later, the HPCSA, which governs the medical professions in South Africa, charged Tim with violating medical ethics by giving allegedly unconventional professional advice on Twitter, an act it labelled as 'disgraceful conduct'.

Since he hadn't practised for years, he could have avoided the whole thing by resigning his medical commission and they would have had no jurisdiction over him, but instead, he chose to stand his ground. A lot of people were concerned; even his wife apparently turned to him one night while they were driving somewhere and said, 'I'm afraid you might lose.'

'I could,' he said and kept driving, thinking to himself, *If I'm vindicated, though, then the diet is vindicated in the eyes of the public.*

What he thought was going to be one hearing, turned into a multiple hearing ordeal, watched by millions around the world, that lasted three years before he was finally, completely exonerated. The trial is reported to have cost him a lot, but he feels it was totally worth it.

Sir Isaac Newton, the famous English scientist, once said, 'If I have seen further, it is by standing on the shoulders of giants.' We all get to stand on the shoulders of Professor Timothy Noakes so that we can see further.

It sets a precedent, right? It's like the legal thing where lawyers cite precedent. They can say this thing happened back in the day, and this is what those judges found in that case. And that carries a lot of weight legally. Whenever there's a controversy of some kind, like when people are threatened with losing their jobs for advocating

TCR to their patients, there's this trial to go back to. It set a precedent and is like the linchpin on which people often base their defence. We are all very grateful to him for having stood his ground and enduring that ordeal in order to get the truth out.

Skipping forward a bit more, we get to meet another giant. Pam and I went to visit my family, who had all moved; everyone except me had moved to Perth, Australia. I became aware of an orthopaedic surgeon named Gary Fettke, who lives on the island of Tasmania, a part of Australia located roughly south of Melbourne. We saw a bunch of videos he put out and really liked his personality and what he was teaching, so we thought that while we were in Perth, we would just hop across to Tasmania and do an interview with him, which I could put on our YouTube channel.

It was a hell of a lot more than a 'hop' to get across there via Melbourne from Perth, I can tell you that for free. I had everything set up with a hotel in Launceston and a rental car on my points, and I reached out beforehand to his wife, Belinda, to ask her for an address to put into the GPS when we got there.

'Nonsense,' was her reply. 'Cancel all that. You're coming to stay with us. What time does your flight get in so that I can pick you up at the airport?'

We arrived around lunchtime on Friday. Gary came home from work that evening, and they dropped us back off at the airport on Sunday night to catch our flight home. We literally didn't stop talking for two and a half days. It was just the most amazing experience.

One of the main reasons that I had wanted to go and talk to him was the fact that he had run into very similar problems to Tim Noakes and had been reported to his board by a dietitian in his hospital for giving nutritional advice to some of his patients. I wanted to talk with him about that, but he also had an incredible personal story of his own that warrants telling first.

He was diagnosed with a benign but aggressive pituitary tumour in 2000, which required surgery to debulk the tumour, as well as radiotherapy and chemotherapy – they were unable to remove the tumour at the time.

After 11 years of intermittent chemotherapy, it was recommended by a pharmacist that he consider including metformin as an adjunct therapy because of an unexpected side effect of the drug in trials showing less incidence of cancer and even a remission of cancer in the group taking metformin compared to those who weren't.

He was on so many medications already that he thought, *No, I just can't take another one.* So he started investigating what metformin actually does. And it turns out that it's a type 2 diabetes drug that lowers the blood glucose level. So what they were prescribing for him was an off-label use for it, so he thought, *Well, if it's going to lower the sugar in my blood, then why don't I just not eat sugar?* So he literally stopped eating sugar, and everything changed for him.

What was quite fortuitous for us was that after Belinda picked us up at the airport, we were driving around to get groceries for the weekend, and he actually called her. She answered on the car phone so we could all hear. He had just got the results of his post-annual MRI. So, she answered the phone, and he said, 'No growth!' He and Belinda were excited because that meant no need for more chemo/surgery at the time!! His dietary changes had put the tumour into remission. It was quite a privilege to be able to witness that.

After improving his own health with simple dietary changes, he began to think about how these same changes could improve health outcomes for his patients and the implications of what he had discovered might hold for them. He told us 'back in the day, I had one or two patients (maybe) in a year who would present with non-healing diabetic foot ulcers requiring an amputation of their lower leg. Now it feels like every week there's at least one person requiring amputation of their toes/feet or even lower leg in Northern Tasmania.'

He started studying more and came to see that there was a lot more to it than just sugar. He came across LCHF and has come to coin the phrase 'Low Carb-Healthy Fat' instead of 'High Fat', since he feels it is important to make that distinction. He believed patients with non-healing wounds and uncontrolled blood sugars needed to have animal protein and healthy fats. He made a handout for his patients with some generic basic instructions, and he told me once that he used to advise them to cut out sugar and reduce processed food and instead try to eat two eggs and a piece of cheese. And it was working. His patients were responding, their diabetic ulcers were receding, and he was having to amputate fewer limbs.

Effectively, he was preventing people from having to have their feet cut off. I remember, I think it was the first time that we were there, that he was talking about it he said, 'You know, when you think of hearing about a person having to have a foot amputated, you think about the fact that there is a stump now where the foot used to be and they have to deal with that. But what most people don't think about is the surgeon and the staff who are performing that surgery. There is a nurse who has to hold out a bucket to catch the limb after it is cut off. The sound of that limb falling into the bucket haunts me,' he said. My thought is that it's like a stark reminder of what just happened there. That little story has stuck with me since then.

But somehow, some young dietician was livid that he, as a doctor, had no right to give patients nutritional advice because that's how it is. Doctors don't get trained in nutrition. Nutritionists and dieticians are supposed to be the only ones who can tell them what to eat.

So she reported him to AHPRA, the Australian association that *allegedly* protects people from practitioner misconduct, although, as you will see next, the chances that she was manipulated into reporting him are strong.

Here's the kicker. Belinda had been doing a bunch of research to try to understand why Gary was being targeted so brutally. In November 2018, through her efforts, Gary was given access to a vexatious, unsubstantiated 845-page submission to AHPRA that was collated by the Director of Medical Services, on behalf of the Tasmanian Health Service (THS). The same Director of Medical

Services who was posting defamatory material about Gary on a Facebook hate page around the same time. Not only did the Director of Medical Services collate the extensive submission, but he started the submission with the words *'My issues with Dr Fettke are ...'* Within the document, Gary found two letters from the CEO of the Dietitians Association of Australia (the DAA) addressed to the then CEO of the Launceston General Hospital (LGH) effectively demanding that he be *'silenced'*. Incredibly, the CEO of the LGH wrote to the Director of Medical Services, copying three other people and asking, *'Can we push this along to the next level?'* A short time later, Gary was 'conveniently' reported to AHPRA.

They launched a 4 1/2 year Star Chamber investigation into the scope of practice of an orthopaedic surgeon and whether dietary advice fitted into it. Could an orthopaedic surgeon recommend his patients reduce sugar to improve their health outcomes and prevent surgery?

So the people high up in these organisations were trying to have him disbarred from practising. Many people turned on him. We actually saw a picture that Belinda showed to us. Their daughter had a cat, and it used to love to jump up as high as it could and try and catch things. So she used to tease it with a toy of some kind, and it would jump up with his arms spread out and try to catch this toy.

Belinda had taken a picture of it, and Gary took the photo of the family cat to work after the theatre team were encouraged to bring photos of their pets to work for a photo board in theatre. Somebody in the hospital, who he worked with, enlarged that picture, drew a dagger through the middle of the cat and then pasted it up on Gary's locker in the hospital.

Eventually, all allegations and trumped-up charges were dropped, and Gary received a formal apology from the AHPRA medical board in 2018, although the apology was never made public knowledge by AHPRA, and it only showed up 16 months after it was written. I'm sure it still hurts. Ultimately, after all that Gary went through, Australia is now beginning, if not somewhat reluctantly, to recognise

TCR and has included the approach in their best practice guidelines (see Resources section at the end).

One final anecdote here about eggs before I move on. I used to hate eggs. I used to think I was allergic to them because they made me feel ill. I've come to realise that it's the smell and the taste of the eggs that turn my stomach. If anything's got eggs in it, but I can't smell or taste the egg, then I'm fine. As a youngster, my mom was insisting that we eat all these eggs because, before things changed, she was being told that eggs were really good for us, which, it turns out, is true. She was insisting that I eat eggs, even though they made me feel ill. I forget when it was, but at some point, I was old enough to stand up and say, 'No, I'm not eating these.'

It really bummed Pam out as well. She loves eggs, but she couldn't cook them in the house because I would freak out. There was this time when we were going to Pam's folks for Easter dinner one year and I was training for Comrades, so I ran from our home to their house while Pam drove ahead. It was about 20 miles, so I was pretty tired and sensitive when I got there. When I walked into the house, they were busy making deviled eggs, so the whole house was permeated with the smell of eggs. I turned green, did an about-turn, and ran out of the house. Pam felt so bad that she had forgotten about my issue with eggs, and I felt terrible for reacting the way that I did. They opened all the windows and doors and opened and closed the oven where the ham was cooking. Pam was feverishly cutting up oranges to get rid of the smell before I could finally go back in.

Anyway, we were staying with Gary and Belinda in their beautiful home in Tasmania, where they have chooks (chickens) and sheep running around on this huge property. So, on the first morning at breakfast, Gary proudly brings out these beautiful eggs from his chooks, and I have to explain to him that I am not able to eat eggs. So he says, 'What? You don't eat eggs; what are you talking about? I'm going to make you some eggs that you'll eat.'

So he made up these scrambled eggs, put a ton of cheese in them, and he put the plate down in front of me, and I ate them. Pam's eyes were like saucers. She couldn't believe what she was seeing. But we couldn't replicate that at home, and it took a couple of years to figure out that the secret was in the fact that Belinda had cooked bacon before Gary had cooked the eggs, and he had even put some chopped bacon in the eggs themselves. It turns out that the smell of cooking bacon neutralises the smell of the eggs, and putting some bacon in the eggs hides their taste. That was why I was able to eat them.

So now I'm able to eat eggs, that's huge! It's a big rigmarole because we have to cook a bunch of bacon and chop it up into little pieces and grate a bunch of cheese, but I can eat eggs now, and the discovery goes back to the chooks in Tasmania for which I owe Gary, and the chooks, a debt of gratitude.

We all get to stand on Gary's shoulders too! But with both these stories, I get ahead of myself.

CHAPTER 8

THE FIRST EVENT

After six months on this voyage of discovery, everything had changed for me. My weight came down to what I used to call my fighting weight back when I was running all these ultra-marathons. The respiratory issues I had been dealing with for as long as I can remember cleared up. I felt great. My chronically aching knees weren't hurting anymore, and I was loving running again.

I was kind of wondering how it was that I had not even heard of a ketone before, you know, up until six months previously. And I just felt driven, obliged even, to try to help other people like me who had never heard about ketones to actually learn about the diet so that it could change their lives too.

On my birthday in January of 2016, we went out for dinner with our work colleagues. It had got to the stage where it was like, *the first rule of keto is don't talk about keto*. They were so sick of hearing us talk about it all the time, how amazing it was – they thought it was rubbish. But it got to the point in the evening when they had all left, and it was just Pam and me in the restaurant, so we started talking about it.

We had learned from a couple of small conferences. One was held in Australia, called Low Carb Down Under, where I watched some videos to gather what knowledge I had up until then. Another was organised in South Africa. There were also a few smaller ones in the US, with no more than a hundred attendees. I found myself pounding my fist saying, 'We need to put a thousand people in a room.' We needed to organise an event and get a thousand people there. It was ridiculous that I hadn't known about ketones until now. The next day, while Pam was still in bed, I started thinking about it. We had a lot of experience putting on events in the job we were working at the time (or at least I thought I did), so I thought, *Let's do it.*

But I didn't know anybody in the low-carb space. I'd never been to one of these other little conferences. I hadn't been in contact with any of these well-known speakers and researchers who were on YouTube and other platforms on the internet.

I just didn't know any of them. I started looking up speakers who I had seen on the Low Carb Down Under videos. There was one guy who was very prominent at the time, and I reached out to him through his social media. I found Jeff Volek, PhD, MD, a very prominent registered dietitian and scientist, and Stephen Phinney, MD, PhD, a very prominent physician and scientist. I had read their books *The Art and Science of Low Carbohydrate Living*, and *The Art and Science of Low Carbohydrate Performance*, when I was first doing my research on ketones, and the ketogenic diet.

I just looked them up on their websites and sent an email to them. I looked up Gary Taubes as well, an investigative journalist who was most famous, at the time, for his book *Good Calories, Bad Calories* (he's written a few others before and since then). He was, and still is, an icon in this space.

I was thinking that I wanted to put on a conference in San Diego where I lived at that time; *summer, vacation destination, what could be better?* I asked if they would be interested in appearing and speaking. The one guy basically came back straight away, and he ended up helping to put me in contact with a bunch of people saying, 'Hey, if you're looking for speakers, here are some people to contact.'

Jeff Volek came back and said he would do it. Actually, I lie, it took him a while because the email they had on his site was wrong. It was months down the line before I finally got a hold of him and signed him up.

Steve Phinney asked if I had any money to put in to fund some research instead of putting on this event. Unfortunately for him, that was absolutely not the case. He didn't actually end up coming to speak at our first event, but he's spoken at many of them since then.

But the big thing, the turning point, I think, was Gary Taubes. He got back to me and said, 'Hey, can we have a chat about this?' I ended up on a call with him, and I was very aware of what his time was worth to him so I was trying to kind of get through it really quickly. I often tell this story when I introduce him at the events and say it was like I had asked to marry his daughter or something.

But in the end, we talked for about an hour. By the end, he seemed to be confident enough that I knew what I was doing and so he said to me, 'Okay, if you do this, I'll come and speak.' I was on speakerphone, and Pam was standing off to the side, down the corridor and listening in. I hung up the phone and looked at her and said, 'Shit, this is real. We have to put on a conference now.'

That was the moment when I realised that we were actually going to do this.

He's been such an amazing supporter of ours ever since then and has spoken at many of our events. I hung up the phone and chatted with Pam for a bit and then went back to work. It might not have been exactly the very next email I opened, but that's my memory of it; it was from a colleague of ours from the business that we were working in at the time who'd become a really good friend of ours. He had this app that would insert a random famous quote at the end of his signature block. The one at the bottom of his email, in this case was a quote from Winston Churchill, which you will have seen on the back cover of this book:

'There comes a certain moment in everyone's life,
a moment for which that person was born.
That special opportunity, if he seizes it,
will fulfil his mission, a mission for which he is
uniquely qualified. In that moment,
he finds greatness. It is his finest hour.'

You can't make this stuff up! It certainly gave me some added inspiration to get on and do this thing, but when I look back on it now, it is so much more meaningful. With 22 LowCarb*USA* events under our belts (and a 23rd coming up around the time this book will hopefully be published), the establishment and growth of our nonprofit, the Society of Metabolic Health Practitioners (which you will hear about later) and all the amazing things that have transpired since then, I look back on the moment when I read that quote and I don't quite know about finding greatness, but it was definitely my finest hour.

So we decided to do this event in San Diego. We started looking around for hotels. We didn't have a conference coordinator; we didn't even know people like that existed. I don't remember exactly how we were searching for hotels, I think I just Googled 'hotels in downtown San Diego' and started contacting them and saying, 'I'm looking at putting on a conference in July and asking if they had availability.'

July was six months away, I don't know what I was thinking, but we were trying to put it on in July. We had no social media presence. We had no website. We had nothing. We just started building all of that up from scratch while trying to find a hotel at the same time.

We were greenhorns, and it was like this hotel saw us coming. We had no idea what we were doing. I thought we had experience organising events, but it turned out we were only handling the arrangements. I had never dealt with the contracting side and had no idea how much of a nightmare it could be. We ended up signing a contract with this hotel that was totally outrageous. Since we were planning to put a thousand people in the room, I was thinking a thousand people times [X] amount for the ticket price. That will easily cover any of our expenses. But I came to find out that putting a thousand people in the room is not as easy as I thought and you have to give a lot of discounts to sell the tickets you do sell.

When you sign a contract like this with a hotel, you have two options: You can either pay a rental fee for the meeting space or you can commit to a contracted room block and a minimum food and beverage (F&B) spend. You basically order dinner or some kind of meal. But there's a minimum amount that you need to spend to cover the facility rental.

For the room block, they give you a slightly discounted price on the rooms, but you still have to sell all of them, with a little attrition allowance built in. And if you don't, you're on the hook for the ones that you don't sell. We had no idea what a risk it was committing to that contract, actually signing something that said we were going to sell 500 rooms and pay $100,000, or whatever it was, in minimum F&B. We're on the hook for that now.

Then there was also a deposit schedule. So we had to pay an initial deposit, and then starting a month later and monthly throughout the build-up to the event, we had to pay in more and more money towards this minimum amount that we were committed to pay. But we weren't getting the ticket sales. We were way behind what I was kind of naively expecting to sell. We didn't have the money to pay these deposits. And what also came up when the first bill arrived, like a month later, was that when they quote you, say, $100,000 minimum F&B, that is $100,000++. I didn't even notice the '++', and I had no idea what it even meant.

What that means is that it's $100,000 plus a 25% service fee, plus sales tax on that total. So effectively, it adds about 35% to your original quote. Your quote for $100,000 is now $135,000 in terms of your real cost.

I also got in touch with the audio/visual guys, their in-house A/V people. We were planning a three-day event at that stage. They came back with a quote to do the A/V. I'm thinking, *A/V is like you've got this little projector and a screen and, you know, a couple hundred bucks.* $60,000 was the quote for the A/V and I literally had a heart attack. I just couldn't believe it – oh, and that's $60,000++, so it's really $81,000.

So at this stage, I'm literally not going to be able to do this. If there's no way I can even pay the deposits the hotel was expecting, how am I going to afford another $81,000 for the A/V?

Luckily, our contract said that we were allowed to bring in external A/V people. We didn't have to use their super expensive in-house folks. I found someone who was probably half of that (and no ++). I also got in touch with a guy called Dr Andreas Einfeldt, who was in Sweden and had started an organisation called Diet Doctor, where he provided really high-quality videos to teach people about this diet. Did I mention that the $60,000++ didn't include recording the event either? That was going to be another exorbitant cost to get somebody to actually film it.

Andreas agreed to come out from Sweden and film the event and he agreed to pay half of the A/V cost as well. In return, he would be able to use the videos on his site.

He agreed to share them with me, and I could provide them to our attendees as well. That was how I was coping with that bomb-shell. However, around a month to three weeks before the event, the hotel representatives were really stomping their feet, saying, 'We need this money!' We just didn't have it.

Our credit cards were now maxed out and any money that we were collecting from ticket sales was being used to pay down some of these credit cards in order to pay what we could on the next bill from the hotel and max out the cards again.

We only had a small bandwidth on our new business credit card so this was mainly on my personal credit cards. We just kept paying the hotel what we could as we paid those cards down. We eventually arranged to meet with the hotel manager.

You know how you have these things in your life that you can look back on and still see them vividly? This is one of them. I remember sitting in the hotel lobby, I mean he didn't even take us to his office or a meeting room. We were literally sitting in the lobby of the hotel, and he was saying, 'Look, we need these payments.' and I was telling him, 'Well, look, we don't have the money.'

At that stage, we had about 300 people signed up already. 300 people were coming from all over the country and from a bunch of different places around the world as well: Sweden, South Africa, Malaysia, the UK. One person had even signed up from the Czech Republic (we'll get to that later). I said, 'There are people coming from all over the world and we have taken money from them, but we've given you all the money that we've collected from them, so I can't pay them back if we cancel this now. You're not going to give me that money back, are you? We can't pay these people back. What the hell were we going to do?' I was almost in tears.

I don't even remember exactly what else I said or how I managed to get him to come around. I just basically said something to the effect of, 'Look, we're still pounding away. We're expecting to sign up a bunch more people. And, you know, even if we have to borrow the money later, we'll find a way to pay this bill. But we cannot cancel. We just can't.' I don't know how, but he agreed.

So we went ahead with the event. We showed up at the hotel the day before to set everything up. Again, I've never done this before. Well, we've done an event before, so I knew how the registration and stuff works, but we had never really set up the room. It was kind of done for us before we got there at the ones we had done before (again, I was realising that I didn't know as much about events as I thought I did). The A/V guys were supposed to be coming in that morning. However, they had a breakdown. They were coming down from LA and their truck broke down. They arrived late in the afternoon.

Then we found out that the service elevators at the back of the hotel were broken. The A/V team had to come around the front and literally bring all their equipment through the revolving doors at the front of the hotel and carry it up the stairs in the lobby to the ballroom that was up on the landing. They carried all their equipment up there and started setting it up.

By the time it got to the day before the event, we had sold about 350 tickets. The plan was to have an early registration from about 5 to 7 and then go to dinner. We had a few friends helping us at the registration desk who weren't even low-carb people, they were just friends of ours who agreed to come and volunteer to help us. They were pretty amazed at what we were actually doing.

Because the A/V guys were so late, they were still setting up late into the night, and I needed to be there to oversee them do that. So one of our volunteers, Sara Cates, basically decided to go into town to get us all something to eat. There were a lot of restaurants and takeaway places that were sort of within easy walking distance from this hotel so she took a walk.

She came back and said, 'You can't believe what's going on. There are people in the streets everywhere, running around and jumping up and down. It's like, craziness out there.'

The attendees at our event were thrilled to have the opportunity to meet their heroes – people who had written influential books, conducted important research, shared insights about their clinical work with patients, and who had changed these attendees' lives. Now they were going to get a chance to see them in the flesh and even get a chance during the Q&A to maybe even ask them a question or two. It was astounding.

I hadn't seen it personally, but Sara's description of what she had witnessed in the streets was really inspiring. And it stuck with us. It's kind of one of the main reasons, I think, that we ended up agreeing to, or deciding to, keep moving forward and do another one when the idea came up.

So we did the event. There were a lot of things that weren't very well organised, mainly because I didn't know any better. But they weren't major showstoppers. It was just stuff that could have been organised better. With all the events since then, we've fixed those things.

Having had a lot less experience than we thought we had, I think it went really well. And the excitement in the expos in the evenings was palpable. We had Dry Farm Wines there with their sugar-free wine, and they were doing a wine tasting outside during the expo before the dinner. I remember being in the main hall, packing everything up and sorting everything out, shutting down for the day, and then going through into that expo area.

It was just humming. It was amazing. I just stood there and looked at it and thought, *Pam and I did this!* It was absolutely incredible what we had managed to do and, like a duck swimming serenely on top of the water, no one saw the frantic paddling that had been going on under the water so that we could be standing there.

It was during that first evening in the expo, when people were coming up to us and saying, 'When's the next one?'

I looked at them and said, 'This is it. We only planned to put this one event on.'

They said, 'No, no, you need to have another one next year, and we'll buy the tickets now!

'We don't even know who will be presenting or anything,' we said.

'We don't care,' they responded excitedly, 'If it's anything like this, we're coming back!'

At that stage, I'd made these promises to the hotel manager that we would get them paid, but I didn't have the money. So it suddenly occurred to me that, *Hey, you know what? If we have an event next year and we sell early bird tickets to all these people, or at least a bunch of these people here who want to come back next year, maybe that's a way to collect some money in the short term to pay the hotel.* I asked everybody from the stage, 'If we did this, we wouldn't know right now who the speakers would be, but if we did something similar, would you guys buy tickets now to come back next year if we give you a big discount?'

And they all said, 'Yes, of course.'

So I stayed up through Saturday night and built a third page on my website (did I tell you that our first website that got us to that event was only two pages?) for another event, sort of at the same time the next year. We ended up selling 84 tickets, and that got us out of the hotel. Now we'd sold 84 tickets for next year, right? But all the money that we had collected went straight to the hotel for this event. We got home, and there was still one speaker whose expenses I hadn't managed to pay yet. I was going to die before I didn't pay him. We had one vendor who had agreed only to pay us half of the vendor fee upfront, and they were going to pay us the other half afterwards. When I finally managed to get that payment, I was able to pay the speaker what I owed him.

So I paid my part of the A/V, I paid the hotel, I paid everything, but I was completely maxed out on my credit cards. Now we had to find a way to put on another event the next year. By that time, Pam and I had both been forced to step away from the previous job that wasn't really paying us anyway, just from a time perspective, so we had no other source of income. I literally didn't have enough money to pay our rent.

So for the next couple of months, we were able to buy some food, but I didn't pay the rent. One day, I went to get some groceries and when I returned, there was an eviction notice nailed to the door. We didn't know what to do. One of the vendors who had been at the event had approached us and said that we needed to do another one on the East Coast. Actually, a lot of people had come to us and told us we needed to do one on the East Coast. We said, 'No, we can barely do one here in San Diego, let alone one on the East Coast as well.'

But this guy had connections there and it's a long story, but we eventually decided that if we planned something in January in what turned out to be West Palm Beach, then we could start selling tickets to that and maybe start refilling the coffers again. We planned a Florida event really quickly and started selling tickets. We got a good spurt of ticket sales in the beginning, and because of that, we were able to pay enough of our rent so that they were prepared to take the eviction notice down. Over time, we eventually managed to stay in that house. Whatever it was that convinced me, or persuaded me to keep going, I don't know. Why did I think that carrying on and doing another one of these was a good idea? I suppose I felt like it was my mission somehow. It just didn't occur to me that I shouldn't carry on, and I'd taken a bunch of money from people for next year's event (actually two events now). I couldn't exactly just give that back to them, so I couldn't cancel.

So we went and did one in Florida in January 2017, and then we came back to San Diego in July where we did another one, this time with an event management company to help us find a much better contract in a different hotel. Now we've done others throughout the country. We did one in San Francisco and Seattle and even one in Jakarta, Indonesia, but those have been once off and San Diego and Florida have turned out to be our annual events.

At the time of writing this, we've done 22 events. But if I look back at the first one, there are three things that really stand out to me in terms of super positive outcomes from what we had done that weekend.

The first one was a group. There was a lady who lived literally just up the road from where we were living at the time, and she was part of this group where either they, or their child, was suffering from McArdle's disease, which is a glycogen storage disease. In our bodies, some of the sugar and the carbohydrates that we eat get stored in our muscles and our liver as glycogen. That's what our body turns to for producing energy when we move about and go through our day (this refers to people whose metabolisms have not adapted to run on ketones, just to be clear). These people with McArdle's don't have any glycogen stored at all. So when they try to get up, they literally can't. It's a debilitating disease.

There are strategies that they have developed to produce what they call a second wind. They rest for a bit, and then they're able to move enough to go to the toilet and do small tasks. But they literally are not able to function. They get a lot of muscle damage from the fact that they're putting stress on the muscles without the energy for the muscles to actually support that effort.

It's a massive thing. There was a group of about six of them who came to this event because they had discovered that if they went on this very strict ketogenic diet, their bodies started running on ketones. They weren't running on glucose anymore. They were then able to function normally, or relatively normally. There's a huge worldwide McArdle's fraternity. And they were getting absolutely hammered by others in that group, chastising them about doing this.

There were the doctors threatening to basically report them for child abuse for putting their children on this diet or even wanting to put their children on this ketogenic diet. They came to our meeting to try and learn more and see if there was a way that they could persuade their community that this was a legitimate option in trying to manage this disease. I gave them five minutes. They all got up on the stage and talked quickly about their disease and how difficult it was for them as they were basically ostracised within their own community for trying to do this, especially with their kids.

Dr Eric Westman was one of the speakers who was at that event. Emily McGuire was a nutritionist from the UK who was also there as a speaker for us. Eric basically instigated this whole effort to help them. He reached out to Emily and two of the folks who were part of this group of attendees, Stacey Reason and Richard Godfrey. The four wrote a paper published in the *Journal of Rare Disorders, Diagnosis and Therapy*. It was called 'Can a Low-Carb Diet Improve Exercise Tolerance in McArdle's Disease?'[1] It was basically a case study and they looked at three cases. Just take a look at the last sentence in the discussion on the first case, '*Overall, he has more energy, no longer worries about keeping up with others, and enjoys being able to play sports without suffering muscle pain afterwards.'* How incredible is that?

If you look at the end of case two, *'She is regularly followed by a healthcare team in Stockholm. Her parents have indicated that this low-carbohydrate ketogenic diet has resulted in a return to normal life.'* That's amazing.

The third one says, *'She is being monitored regularly by her primary care practitioner. She states that she really doesn't suffer any longer, other than if she engages in prolonged anaerobic activities, such as heavy lifting.'*

These three cases document the results in much more detail than that, obviously.

They state at the end of the paper that these are just three cases. It's not a clinical trial or anything, but here are three cases that show that this intervention is something that people should at least take seriously and consider trying. Now, if doctors want to come and try and report them for child abuse, they can point a court to this document that will basically support them. None of this would have happened if those folks had not come to that event and they had not had five minutes to speak on the stage.

I base all my recent events' themes these days on a talk by Admiral Bill McRaven. He speaks about the ten things you can do to change the world. At the beginning of his talk, he makes a significant point: *one person can change the world by giving people hope.*

The next story is about Pavla Hlavicková, who came from the Czech Republic. She is such a tremendous person. I've used her story a couple of times on stage in my later events when talking about the ripple effect. When we manage to inspire one person, we can never know how far that influence might reach. She attended our first event in 2016. A year after she had been at the event, she wrote about it on our Facebook page. I think we were literally getting ready to drive down to the hotel to set up for the 2017 event when we saw it. I read it exactly as she wrote it, hoping that people can almost visualise, or hear, her saying it.

Hi Everyone,

I'd like to share my low carb story with you. It has been almost four years since I heard about lowcarb/ketogenic WOE [Way Of Eating] for the first time. I was fascinated and changed my diet right away with incredible results. I have started to study more to understand better. I am from Prague, Czech Republic, and there is only a few information [sic] about lowcarb in Czech. But I wanted to share my story and my results with other people and motivate them to think more about their diet. That is why I became Nutrition Specialist in 2016. In summer 2016, I have noticed that there was going to be a Low Carb conference in San Diego. Even San Diego [sic] is 10,000 miles from Prague, I knew this was a MUST SEE/HEAR event for me. The conference was such an inspiration for me that I have started my Lowcarb food blog in September 2016. In January 2017 I have founded a Czech FB Lowcarb group with only a few members. [Now she posted this on Aug 31st, 2017, 8 months after starting the group. She goes on to say:] I am very proud that I can say we are expecting to reach 10,000 members this Sunday! 1 member for 1 mile from Prague to San Diego last year.

Thank you, Pam Devine and Doug Reynolds, for being such an inspiration to me.'

I still struggle with that and choke up every time I read it. We checked in with Pavla recently and at the time of writing this book, she was about to hit 200,000 followers in her Facebook group. That's 200,000 people in the Czech Republic who are being trained and being exposed to this information because of one person who came to our event.

This was actually the next year, in San Diego in 2017. Dr Brian Lenzkes was an attendee and he actually had a practice just up the road from the hotel. He had seen that this event was going on and that continuing education credits were available for doctors. So he thought, *Hey, why not attend and see about this?* Now, he had been reading about fasting from Jason Fung and a little bit about low carb before this. Because he had been struggling with his weight and his health following the same advice that he was giving to his patients, he had been trying some ideas out on himself, very much like we did when we started – you don't want to tell anybody about it, like under the radar.

But he started to lose weight and people were saying to him, 'Hey Doc, what's going on? You're looking so much better.' I think he just fobbed them off, saying he was trying another diet or something. He didn't want to admit to them, or explain to them, what he was doing at the time.

Then he came to our event and he saw all these amazing doctors and scientists giving these talks and speaking about it. He thought to himself, *Wow, this is really legit. This is not just a fad thing that I should be following clandestinely.*

The need for doctors like him who understand and embrace these ideas is huge. During the event, he got a phone call from his receptionist in his practice saying, 'What the hell are you doing?'

And he said, 'What's wrong?'

She said, 'Our switchboard is blowing up. We got so many people phoning in trying to get an appointment.' All that he had done was stand up at the microphone for the Q&A and say, 'Hi, my name is Dr Brian Lenzkes, and I'm a physician. My practice is literally just up the road here in San Diego.'

There were people in the audience from San Diego who were so desperate to find a doctor who understood low-carb or who was at least open to it. They all went outside and started looking him up and phoning his office to try and get an appointment to see him.

Then he reached out to me in November of that year; I hadn't even met him at the event. I didn't know him at all. But he wrote to me and said, *'Hey, Doug, is there any chance that we could meet? I'm really inspired by all of this to try to help other people.'*

Of course I agreed, and he drove up and we met at some barbecue rib place. We were sitting there talking and he said, 'You know, I went back to my practice after the event and I didn't start preaching about low carb, but now, when people asked me what I was doing, why I looked so much healthier, and why I had lost so much weight, I would tell them what I was doing. 'It's not conventional, but if you are interested in trying it, I am happy to support you with it.' He created a big folder with links to watch videos and just all this stuff to help people embrace this lifestyle if they wanted to.

He told us, 'You know, in 20 years of practice, I have never had anybody with type 2 diabetes come off insulin. We've all been told that it's a chronic, progressive disease.'

What happens with most people is that you keep increasing the insulin as time goes by. A few of them (actually a lot of them) down the road end up with all sorts of other side effects like neuropathy, or they end up being sent to surgeons like Gary Fettke (who we talked about earlier) to have their lower limbs amputated because of diabetic foot ulcers.

He said that in the four months after the event, he had had 11 patients come off insulin. That is just the most astounding thing to me. So he, like me, felt he should get out there and tell people about it.

He was a member of a very big church locally in San Diego. He went to the pastor and asked him if he would mind if he put on an event. He basically got a couple of people in to speak each day. He spoke a lot himself and taught people about low-carb and the ketogenic diet. He did it for six weeks every Sunday. But there were a lot of people who wanted to actually go to church instead of attending his talk. So he repeated it again each Monday night.

He had 200 people coming every week for six weeks at those two different events. There was a bit of overlap; I think some people came twice, but there were almost 400 people in total to whom he was speaking. We didn't have anything to do with it. We didn't put it on. We didn't even help him. We didn't do anything. We often talk about standing at the back like proud parents, watching this happen, this guy who we had been able to influence at our event.

On the very last Monday night, he had a panel on the stage and I did take part in that. It was a big theatre-type auditorium. Everybody was up in their seats and we were sitting on the stage. We were there for an hour and a half or so. The security guys were peeping in and trying to sort of let us know that we needed to shut things down. So we closed it down, but we all ended up sitting on the edge of the stage, with our legs hanging over the edge. All these people came down from their seats and kind of crowded around us. There was this huge conversation going on because everybody was talking at once.

Brian was talking and I was being asked questions, and Pam was being asked questions. There was more than one person saying something to the effect of, 'Thank you for making my husband [or wife] a better person. Since they started doing this, it has changed them completely.'

People were telling us, 'Hey, I've been doing this. I've been eating so many eggs now, and I've lost this amount of weight. We heard so many stories sitting around there. And the excitement was just contagious.

This was another really proud moment for us. Brian got hold of Jason Fung, who I mentioned before. He was a very well-known advocate of fasting. He also reached out to Dr Tro Kalayjian, and the three of them started a podcast. It's called *The LowCarbMD Podcast*. Jason bowed out at some point, and with the two of them, it is now one of the top podcasts in the space.

I think they hit a million downloads within their first year of launching it. Brian and Tro have literally reached millions of people just because Brian came to our event. So that's pretty stunning, I reckon.

At the time of this writing, we just finished our 22nd event, which was in San Diego.

Next year's San Diego event (2025) will be at a very nice new property on Coronado Island. That's going to be for our 10th anniversary – our 10th annual San Diego event since we started this whole thing. As I mentioned, we did one in San Francisco, we've done one in Seattle, and we've done a couple of one-day events, including one in Brainerd Lakes, MN, this year.

We've been kind of living in that financial hole we had created for ourselves before the first event. Basically we collect money for an event and pay down the credit cards. Then we put the event on, get the bill for the event and basically max out the credit cards.

Over time, we were slowly climbing out of that hole. Each year after the event, we would pay the event off and the cards weren't quite fully maxed out anymore.

We were slowly going to get to a point one day where we wouldn't have any credit card debt at all. And then we had a disastrous year in 2019. We had contractually overcommitted to two different events – both the Florida event and the San Diego event – for all sorts of reasons.

We had a special Latino day at the Florida event – an extra day on the Monday afterwards – specifically for the Latino community. We hired a translation company to provide real-time translations, allowing the audience to listen via headphones. If the presenter spoke in English, a Spanish translation was provided; for English speakers, a translation was given when the presentation was in Spanish. A couple of things contributed to the problem there.

First of all, in order to secure the meeting hall for another day, we had to commit to 100 extra room nights. We were kind of hoping to get 100 people there so we signed the contract. We ended up getting about 100 people there, however, none of them came and stayed in the hotel. Many drove through the night to be there in the morning, but not one person booked a room. So we were on the hook for those 100 room nights (well, 80 after the allowable attrition).

The second problem was there was a huge storm in the area on the Sunday and the airport was shut down. Many folks who had been there through the weekend at our main event couldn't get home. They had to stay in the hotel on the Sunday night as well – which we didn't get credit for – by the way. We arranged food for all the staff and speakers who were staying over and a few attendees who had come for the weekend but were staying for the Latino Day as well. But they served it in the same dining area as we had used for the dinners during the main event. Somehow, the weekend attendees who were stuck in the hotel because of the storm noticed these dinners going on and they thought, *Oh, there's a Sunday night dinner as well.* So they all came and tucked in and the hotel ran out of food. The chef was freaking out, and they kept coming out and counting all the people seated at the tables and the headcount was way higher than the number I'd given them. So when we got the bill, there was a massive penalty on there for that extra food and the 80 room nights.

Then, in San Diego later that year, we got too excited about how fast we were growing and we (actually, I) stupidly signed a contract for way more than the minimum the hotel required for us to secure the space we needed. I should have insisted that we just contract for whatever the minimum requirement was for that space. But I was excited and everything was growing. I just thought, *Yeah, you know, we had 650 people there in 2018. We'll have more than that next year, no problem. Right?* Wrong!

There were a bunch of reasons why that didn't happen, which I won't go into. In the end, we had all these penalties for the minimums that we didn't meet at these two events. The total for the two was $90,000 in extra charges. The hotels are ruthless. They don't care that you're trying to do some good in the world, they just want their money!

So after all that progress that we'd made in starting to climb out of that financial hole, we wound up right back in there again. Even after maxing out the credit cards again, we still didn't have enough money to cover those penalties.

Again, people came to our rescue. Dorian Greenow and Gemma Kochis from Keto Mojo found a way by licensing our videos to put them on their site so that we could take that money and pay off the hotels. We even borrowed money from my parents and Pam's mom. Finally, we managed to pay all those hotel bills. Then 2020 hit, and it was COVID. It hit after Boca, so that event was unaffected. However, we couldn't get into the hotel in San Diego in 2020, so we had to pivot.

I often say that I built this 'Boeing cockpit,' this whole streaming system, in my office at home in San Diego so that we could do a virtual San Diego event, and it was pretty amazing because we got like 800 people to sign up for that.

That's the closest I've ever come to putting a thousand people in the room like I was saying I wanted to do all those years before. We did another virtual one in place of the Boca event in January 2021.

Then we started to climb back out of the hole again. In San Diego, everything opened up in May of 2021. We were now contracted and obliged to have an event in that August. A lot of the people who we had rolled over from the previous event that was cancelled still didn't want to travel, so they didn't come.

When we started selling the tickets in May, sales ramped up, and it went really well. Then the Delta COVID variant hit, and we literally didn't sell one more ticket between then and the event in August when we actually had the event. I think we had about 150 people show up, but it was awesome to see people again. It was awesome that so many people spent money and took the time to come out and be there with us.

I was pretty choked up when I got on the stage at the beginning to kick things off. All I could get out was a choked up, 'You came!' When we brought all the equipment into the hotel a couple of days before, I looked around, and I honestly had no idea if anybody was going to show up. So it was a massive relief to be looking at all these faces.

However, one of the things that we'd learned from COVID was that there was a real need to have a streaming or virtual component. With all the live events we've done since then, we always include a live-streaming component for those who can't attend in person – whether due to financial constraints, time limitations, or other reasons. They can purchase a ticket to watch it live or access the recordings afterwards. Continuing education credits are still available to them for this as well.

So that's kind of been the model going forward. We have a live in-person component, which is slowly growing from the 150 we had after COVID, and each year, we're getting a few more. I think we've got up to the point where we are actually getting about 300 in-person at each event, Florida and San Diego. Then, at least that number again will be on the live stream as well. That's been pretty rewarding.

A few weeks ago, we finished a deal with Dr. Jeff Gerber, who was the guy who put on the low-carb conference in Denver. He is one of the guys who was enormously helpful to us during the first couple of events that we put on. He was struggling to do that event each year and continue his practice. It's just too hard, so we merged and took over that organisation from him.

A lot of people have always thought that the Low Carb Denver conference was part of the LowCarb*USA* stable, but it wasn't. Now it is! We're not going to have an extra event next year (2025), but we're thinking we will do something in the middle of the country at some point. San Diego will still be our flagship event each year, but maybe we're going to alternate the January event. We'll do Florida in 2025 and 2026 (since we already have contracts) and then find a venue in the middle of the country in 2027. I don't think we'll go back to Denver, but maybe something in Texas, where we live now?

CHAPTER 9

THE KETOGENIC DIET

9.1 INTRODUCTION

W e've talked a lot about the ketogenic diet and how effective it can be in combating not just obesity but pretty much all the chronic diseases that plague our society in this day and age. You can see with the nonprofit that we'll talk about a bit later – with the Society of Metabolic Health Practitioners – we've become more and more focused on not just low-carb or the ketogenic diet, but on metabolic health, which may occur independently of weight changes.

There are many factors that contribute to improved metabolic health. In the beginning, it was all about the ketogenic diet. But actually, there's a whole lot more to it than that.

The two biggest contributors, in my opinion, are diet and exercise. This chapter is about the ketogenic diet.

Confusion around the ketogenic diet abounds in the media and on the internet, making it difficult for everyone. This can detract from the fact that more and more healthcare providers are successfully implementing ketogenic or carbohydrate-reduced diets to help people improve their health. At one point, Dr Eric Berg suggested that I publish something on the LowCarb*USA* website to dispel the numerous concerns (myths) that exist about the ketogenic diet.

Once we started to take this seriously, it became clear to us that anything we published on the LowCarb*USA* website needed to be accurate, devoid of hyperbole and dogma, and supported by the literature. So I rewrote the original draft I was provided and then turned to Sarah Rice, whom I hardly knew at all at the time, to ask for help in identifying a few papers that I could reference to support what I was saying, but that just opened up a huge can of worms.

Sarah Rice has put together, in my opinion, the best and most extensive curated database of vetted research papers in the metabolic health space. She was not happy with the accuracy of the language I was using most of the time, and so she started editing it, which turned into rewriting it and even adding a few sections for completeness. The version that is published on the LowCarb*USA* site at the time of writing has a list of 337 references that are cited throughout the document.[2]

This chapter is basically a summary of that document with the intent of describing what the ketogenic diet is, how it came about, answering common questions, and considering the benefits of embracing this dietary and lifestyle intervention. The plan is to publish the full ketogenic diet document as its own book in 2025. Scan the QR code at the end of the book so you can sign up for updates on that publication.

9.2 A BRIEF HISTORY OF THE KETOGENIC DIET

Prior to the development of the ketogenic diet, as we know it, the benefits of therapeutic carbohydrate reduction had already been investigated for the treatment of diabetes mellitus. This condition is one of the oldest recognised diseases with descriptions found in early Greek history (81–138 AD). A clearer description occurred in 1678 from Thomas Willis, where he noted the sweet taste of urine in patients, and the Latin word *mellitus* was added to further describe the condition. Connections between the pancreas, high sugar concentrations, and organ damage took a further 100 years to piece together.[3]

In 1797, Rollo noted that the abnormally high sugar production, which he considered a stomach disorder, could be managed with a diet high in fat and meat. Rollo published cases of two patients with diabetes who were able to be managed in this way, but there was limited uptake of this approach at the time.[4] In these early studies, there was no clear differentiation between type 1 and type 2 diabetes.

One hundred years later, Elliot Joslin found a low-carbohydrate, high-fat dietary approach for the treatment of type 1 diabetes to be successful and published his findings between 1893 and 1928. He recommended the consumption of vegetables with less than 5% carbohydrate and suggested a diet of 70% fat with carbohydrates limited to 10%.[5] At a similar time, Frederick Allen worked on the treatment of diabetes by fasting his patients and adding back different combinations of carbohydrates, proteins, and fat, and measuring this against the amount of sugar he found in their urine. Using this methodical approach, a successful ratio was found to occur at approximately 70% fat and 8% carbohydrate. Allen published his work in 1919 in the form of a series of patient cases.[5] The work of Joslin and Allen demonstrated that dietary changes could influence the blood glucose responses (type 1 and type 2 diabetes) and insulin responses (type 2 diabetes), providing some insight and enabling select patients limited options for managing their condition.

Let us not forget Dr William Harvey, who advised William Banting to adopt a low-carbohydrate approach to treat his obesity in 1862. Banting's subsequent *Letter on Corpulence*, in which he describes how he was able to lose 50 lbs, is one of the first commentaries on this approach to obesity.[6] Well-renowned surgeon Sir William Osler describes a low-carbohydrate approach in his textbook (1892) for the treatment of obesity and diabetes, suggesting 65% fat,

32% protein, and 3% carbohydrate and the removal of fruit and garden produce from the diet.[7,8]

The discovery of insulin by Banting and Best in 1921 revolutionised the management of type 1 diabetes. Initial challenges included difficulties in maintaining adequate supplies, but the first patients received treatment in early 1922. At first, adherence to a high-fat, low-carbohydrate diet in conjunction with the administration of insulin was the standard approach, but in the following decades, a higher-carbohydrate diet became more popular.[9,10]

In 1911, it was noticed that patients with epilepsy who underwent a period of starvation had less severe seizures. In the early 1920s, two researchers began looking at ways to support the production of ketone bodies via dietary approaches rather than starvation, and the ketogenic diet was born. The focus of their research was the production of ketone bodies, hence the name 'ketogenic'.[11] In 1938, the discovery of the first medication for the treatment of epilepsy began to influence the research directions, and over time, the popularity of the ketogenic diet reduced.

The use of the ketogenic diet in medicine has a history dating back hundreds of years. While we can be grateful for medical advances, history reminds us of the power of nutritional approaches for both metabolic and neurological conditions and their potential for success.

9.3 WHAT IS A KETOGENIC DIET?

According to the *Society of Metabolic Health Practitioners* (SMHP™), a well-formulated ketogenic diet includes adequate energy, protein, fat, vitamins, and minerals. The ketogenic diet may be defined by an absolute amount of carbohydrates per day (grams/day):[12,13]

- Very low-carbohydrate ketogenic (VLCK) diets recommend 30g or less of dietary carbohydrate per day.

- Low-carbohydrate ketogenic (LCK) diets recommend 20–50 g of dietary carbohydrate per day.
- Medical ketogenic therapy (MKT) involves a more focused approach in obtaining therapeutic levels of ketones, which may be required for certain conditions like epilepsy, neurological disorders, supporting cancer treatment, and mental health conditions. Dietary carbohydrate intake is < 50 g/day, often in the lower end of the range. Adjustments may be required to facilitate target ketone levels, and an experienced practitioner may be required to guide the process.

Limiting carbohydrates to 20 to 50 grams per day allows the body to enter a state of nutritional ketosis, where the hormone profile mimics a fasted state, promoting the breakdown of fat stores and releasing fatty acids into circulation. These fatty acids are metabolised to ketone bodies (ketones) by the liver and secreted as an alternative fuel source. In addition, glucose is manufactured by the liver via gluconeogenesis. This allows the body to generate sufficient fuel to fulfil its energy requirements.

Some conditions benefit from higher levels of ketone bodies for therapeutic benefit, and this type of ketogenic diet may be referred to as medical ketogenic therapy or similar. Adjustments to macronutrient ratios and measurement of ketones may be required to ensure a therapeutic effect is reached. Many individuals are able to achieve their health goals using a less significant level of carbohydrate reduction, which is where a personalised approach is important.

A zero-carbohydrate (or carnivore) approach is another variation of the low-carbohydrate, high-fat ketogenic diet. While this may seem restrictive, this approach serves as an exclusion protocol, allowing the body to heal. People who find this approach helpful often have autoimmune, inflammatory, gastrointestinal, and mental health conditions. Over time, as the body heals, a wider range of foods may be introduced, and this can include plants if desired.

The ketogenic diet is often referred to as 'keto' in the media, but it is important to measure diet quality and approach against standardised terms to ensure the best chance of achieving desired health outcomes. Over time, different versions of the ketogenic diet have been developed, which introduced options for more flexible approaches in helping people to achieve their health goals. Tailoring the level of carbohydrate reduction to individual health goals can make the approach easier to follow.

9.4 WHY CONSIDER A KETOGENIC DIET?

The ketogenic diet has experienced a surge in interest in recent years, driving the research forward and considering a range of applications. We now have many studies showing low-carbohydrate and ketogenic diets to be safe and effective for a number of conditions, demonstrating metabolic and neurological benefits.

Metabolic changes, driven by a reduced carbohydrate diet, act to regulate various pathways that become dysregulated in our modern food environment, giving rise to chronic disease. While many people are able to reach their health goals using a low-carbohydrate approach, some find the additional benefits of a ketogenic diet more helpful. This is where a personalised approach is important.

9.4.1 METABOLIC CONDITIONS

A ketogenic diet is able to improve metabolic conditions primarily by reducing insulin resistance, a key driver of many chronic conditions. Good metabolic health is related to how well your body processes food and how it stores and uses energy. It occurs when metabolic pathways are operating efficiently without placing stress on the body. It may be defined by the following markers, which indicate metabolic pathways are functioning within a healthy range:[12,14]

- A healthy weight and low abdominal fat (waist circumference <102/88 cm for men/women; waist circumference to height ratio <0.5)
- A healthy blood pressure (SBP <120 and DBP <80)
- Low triglycerides (<150 mg/dL or <1.7 mmol/L)
- A healthy HDL cholesterol level (≥40/50 mg/dL or ≥1.04/1.3 mmol/L for men/women)
- A healthy fasting blood glucose (<100 mg/dL or <5.6 mmol/L)

Reducing carbohydrates in the diet reduces the amount of insulin required to manage blood glucose levels, and sensitivity to insulin improves. This dietary approach has been consistently shown to reduce weight, lower blood pressure, lower triglycerides, improve HDL cholesterol, and lower elevated fasting glucose levels.[15]

The table below lists the main ways that a ketogenic diet can help people achieve their health goals.

Benefits of a ketogenic diet	Mechanisms of action
Improves blood glucose and insulin sensitivity	Reducing carbohydrates in your diet reduces blood glucose, and less insulin is required to keep your blood glucose in the normal range. This improves insulin resistance, a condition where the body becomes insensitive to insulin signalling and insulin levels increase.
Regulates hunger signals	Blood glucose and insulin levels drive other hormones that control our hunger. More stable blood glucose and insulin levels help hunger hormones to normalise, and excessive hunger signals reduce.
Helps with healthy weight loss	The ketogenic diet promotes fat burning and improves hunger while providing essential nutrition. The main focus is on reducing carbohydrates, not calories.

Benefits of a ketogenic diet	Mechanisms of action
Helps with the management of type 2 diabetes (may include remission)	Reducing carbohydrates in the diet (usually to 20–50 g/day) directly impacts and reduces blood glucose levels. Lower blood glucose concentrations reduce the amount of insulin required to bring blood glucose into the healthy range. Over time, the body becomes more sensitive to insulin, and medication can usually be reduced.
Helps with the management of type 1 diabetes	Lower levels of carbohydrates in the diet require lower levels of insulin medication in order to keep blood glucose in the healthy range. In type 1 diabetes, blood glucose is more difficult to control due to all of the pathways that are influenced by the loss of pancreatic function. Some insulin will always be required to manage this condition, but the research and patient experiences suggest that management is easier using a low-carbohydrate approach.
Reverses and helps prevent metabolic syndrome	Normalises the features of metabolic syndrome: • reduces waistline (abdominal obesity) • lowers blood pressure • lowers triglycerides • increases HDL cholesterol • reduces fasting blood sugars
Improves fatty liver (also known as non-alcoholic fatty liver)	Excess carbohydrates in the diet activate pathways that promote fat storage. When peripheral fat stores are at capacity, fat is stored in the liver, leading to elevated liver enzymes and disease. Reducing carbohydrates to ketogenic levels stops fat storage and promotes fat burning, improving fatty liver disease.
Can improve kidney function	Chronic kidney disease is generally a feature of metabolic dysregulation, which may be improved using a ketogenic diet. In genetic conditions (autosomal dominant polycystic kidney disease), early research is showing progression of this disease may slow when a ketogenic diet is adopted.

Benefits of a ketogenic diet	Mechanisms of action
Reduces inflammation	Elevated insulin and fat accumulation around the waist drive an increase in inflammatory pathways. A ketogenic diet reduces inflammation by improving these features and blocking other pathways of inflammation.
Supports a healthy gut	A healthy gut is critical to a healthy body, as the gut lining mediates immune and inflammatory pathways and influences hunger signalling via its connection to the brain. Food processing can introduce irritants and create an imbalance in the microbiome. A well-formulated whole-food ketogenic diet removes grains and other potentially irritating foods, supporting gut health, and improving the microbiome.
Supports immune function	A ketogenic diet suppresses inflammation pathways (specifically via the NLRP3 inflammasome pathway) and improves immune T-cell function

(Table information source[12,13])

Other conditions may be improved via the mechanisms described in the table above. These include:

- Metabolic conditions: reproductive health (e.g., PCOS, hypogonadism), lipoedema and lymphoedema, sleep disorders (e.g., sleep apnoea and disturbances associated with neurological conditions).[2,12]
- Inflammatory and immune conditions: fibromyalgia, osteoarthritis, psoriatic arthritis, and chronic pain. Improvements in skin conditions like psoriasis, acne, and hidradenitis suppurativa (acne inversa) have also been reported. Inflammatory gastrointestinal conditions.[2,12]

9.4.2 Neurological conditions

The metabolic improvements that occur using the ketogenic diet also benefit neurological conditions, but ketone body metabolism has additional benefits with regard to brain health. The history of the ketogenic diet gives clues to this effect. It was the presence of ketones that drove the development of this diet and naming. While epilepsy is a distinct neurological condition, there is considerable overlap between this and other neurological conditions where brain energy metabolism, neurotransmitter dysregulation, neuroinflammation, and insulin resistance play a role in disease processes and symptoms. Another clue to the overlap between epilepsy and other brain disorders is the use of epilepsy medications for conditions like migraine and mental health conditions. As noted in the original research, the production of ketones is a key therapeutic benefit. For neurological conditions, it may be necessary for a higher level of nutritional ketosis to be maintained in order to experience the full benefit (medical ketogenic therapy). Additional support and adjustment of dietary components may be required in order to achieve this to the necessary levels and consistency.

A summary of neurological conditions that may benefit from a ketogenic diet can be found in the table on the next page.

Condition	Mechanisms of action
Neurodevelopmental disorders: Epilepsy, autism spectrum disorders, and attention deficit hyperactivity disorder (ADHD), and can include movement (Tourette syndrome), speech, and language disorders.	Improved brain energy metabolism, neurotransmitter regulation, inflammation, improved metabolic and mitochondrial function, and improved gut health. A ketogenic diet is gluten-free and may be supportive of those with food sensitivities, common in children with neurodevelopmental disorders.
Neurodegenerative disorders: Alzheimer's disease, Parkinson's disease, Huntington's disease and amyotrophic lateral sclerosis (ALS) Has also shown benefit for conditions with an autoimmune component (multiple sclerosis, inclusion body myositis)	Improves brain energy metabolism (via the use of ketone bodies and increased mitochondrial function), decreases inflammation, regulates neurotransmitters, and promotes removal of old and damaged cells (autophagy).
Other neurological disorders: Migraine, traumatic brain injury, post-concussion syndrome	Targets multiple pathways, including stabilising blood glucose levels, reducing inflammation, regulating neurotransmitters, neuroprotection, and increased neurotrophic factors.

(Table information source[2,12])

9.4.3 MENTAL HEALTH CONDITIONS

Our metabolic health is tightly connected to our mood and functional capacity. Metabolic disturbances influence brain energy supply, brain network stability, and neurotransmitter balance. Recent research into these connections has created a new field named 'metabolic psychiatry' where the metabolism of the brain and its response to different metabolic therapies are being investigated.[2,12]

At a basic level, many people notice an improvement in mood and concentration as a natural consequence of adopting a ketogenic diet, even where the primary goal was to improve metabolic health or achieve weight loss. Ketone bodies provide a steady energy supply to the brain and have been shown to improve brain network stability. Conversely, glucose has been shown to have a destabilising effect on these networks.[16]

Ketogenic metabolic therapy for mental health conditions is an area where higher levels of ketone bodies seem to influence the level of benefit experienced. In the same way, sticking consistently to a ketogenic way of eating is important for the best results, and this is one area where the support of an experienced practitioner is essential. The effect of the ketogenic diet on metabolism is significant in the setting of mental health conditions, and medication may need to be adjusted as individuals adapt. This may include a temporary increase or decrease in medications.[17]

9.5 Common questions and misconceptions

The ketogenic diet, first used for epilepsy treatment around 100 years ago, was discovered by clinicians as a way to mimic the biochemistry of fasting, offering a sustainable approach to seizure management. Over time, various variations of the ketogenic diet have been studied to evaluate its clinical effect, considering user tolerance and ease of adherence. It is this aspect that may drive some of the confusion around the ketogenic diet, where a range of versions have been developed. It is important to remember that the precise therapeutic application of the ketogenic diet in managing severe conditions like epilepsy may differ from its use for other conditions or as a preferred way of eating. This section addresses some common questions and misconceptions that can occur in conversations about a ketogenic diet.

9.5.1 Is ketone production caused by starvation?

Ketones do not necessarily reflect a state of starvation, where involuntary calorie deprivation leads to nutrient deficiencies, muscle loss, and organ damage. A well-formulated ketogenic diet can provide a steady energy supply and nutritional sufficiency, which protects muscle mass and supports organ health. The diet does not typically advocate calorie reduction but adjusts the source of calories to predominantly come from fat and protein, minimising carbohydrates. In the absence of carbohydrates, the liver oxidises fatty acids to produce ketones, which are readily used as an energy source. The body can store around 2,000 calories worth of sugar (glycogen) but stores around 130,000 calories in body fat. It is the use of this stored body fat that can help normalise body weight, if that is a goal. The brain can utilise glucose produced by the liver or ketone bodies for fuel. This ability to use ketones for fuel is a sign of metabolic flexibility and metabolic health and was key to human survival in times of food scarcity.

9.5.2 Does the ketogenic diet cause ketoacidosis?

Ketoacidosis and nutritional ketosis are two distinct metabolic states. Ketoacidosis is a rare and potentially life-threatening condition that occurs in type 1 diabetes with insufficient insulin levels and can also occur in type 2 diabetes when the body is under stress, such as from surgery or infections. Ketoacidosis may occur where certain medications disrupt counter-regulatory systems involving insulin, leading to high ketone levels, variable glucose levels, and decreased blood pH levels. In these cases, blood ketone levels may range from 10–25 mmol/L (58–145 mg/dL).

Nutritional ketosis is a controlled metabolic state achieved by carbohydrate reduction using a well-formulated diet, maintaining normal ketone concentrations and maintaining healthy blood pH levels. Blood ketone levels typically range between 0.5 and 3 mmol/L (3–17 mg/dL). For some conditions, a slightly higher ketone concentration may be beneficial, but generally, the concentration remains below 5 mmol/L (29 mg/dL).

9.5.3 DOES A KETOGENIC DIET INCREASE THE RISK OF TYPE 2 DIABETES?

The ketogenic diet is a highly effective intervention for preventing, managing, and even reversing type 2 diabetes. Excessive carbohydrate consumption leads to high blood glucose levels, elevated insulin levels, and insulin resistance, causing various chronic conditions, including type 2 diabetes. Restricting carbohydrates effectively controls blood glucose concentrations and keeps insulin levels low, potentially preventing the onset of type 2 diabetes or reversing the condition. This reduction in blood glucose and insulin concentration may be quite rapid, requiring adjustments to diabetes medications as well as other medications like blood pressure medications.

9.5.4 DOES THE KETOGENIC DIET INCREASE THE RISK OF CARDIOVASCULAR DISEASE?

Concerns about the ketogenic diet and increased risk of cardiovascular disease have arisen largely due to two issues: flawed research by Ancel Keys linking saturated fat to heart disease, which has been refuted multiple times, and the use of cholesterol as an isolated metric of risk.[18] The latest science no longer supports the blanket statement that high cholesterol causes heart disease but considers a range of metabolic parameters to be important in determining risk. Total cholesterol or LDL levels are not good predictors of heart disease, especially in the absence of carbohydrates in the diet.[12] The triglyceride/HDL ratio and the count of small, dense LDL particles are more useful predictors of those at risk of heart disease. Studies show that the ketogenic diet can decrease the triglyceride/HDL ratio, reduce the number of small, dense LDL particles, and so reduce the risk of cardiovascular disease.[15] Risk factors consistently associated with cardiovascular disease include diabetes, metabolic syndrome, hypertension, obesity, and hyperinsulinaemia, which may be reliably improved with carbohydrate reduction.

9.5.5 IS CONSUMING SATURATED FAT ON A KETOGENIC DIET DANGEROUS?

Historically, saturated fats have been criticised for their association with heart disease, while unsaturated vegetable (seed) oils have been promoted as heart-healthy. Recent evidence suggests that the relationship between saturated fats and heart health is more complex than previously thought. Whole foods like full-fat dairy, unprocessed meat, and dark chocolate have a complex food matrix and high nutrient density and are not associated with an increased risk of cardiovascular disease.[19] These foods are very different in composition from highly processed, high-fat foods, which are known to be associated with poor health.

9.5.6 IF THE KETOGENIC DIET IS HIGH IN CHOLESTEROL, IS IT BAD FOR CARDIOVASCULAR HEALTH?

Cholesterol is essential for cell membrane integrity, vitamin D synthesis, bile acid production, and hormone synthesis. The liver produces cholesterol according to body needs, and dietary cholesterol intake is not correlated with blood cholesterol concentrations. There is no consistent association between plasma cholesterol and atherosclerosis, and the US dietary guidelines have removed the limit on dietary cholesterol due to lack of evidence.

9.5.7 DOES A KETOGENIC DIET CAUSE NUTRIENT DEFICIENCIES?

A well-formulated ketogenic diet is nutritionally complete and effective across various age groups.[20] It usually includes animal products that provide high-quality bioavailable nutrients like iron, retinol, B12, selenium, and zinc. Nutrient deficiencies can result from not consuming enough nutrient-dense whole foods, such as a diet that is high in processed foods. High-carbohydrate diets, full of processed foods, confectionery, and soft drinks, carry a risk of nutrient deficiencies even in the context of sufficient calories. A target of 1.2 to 2.0 g/kg of body weight is suggested for optimal protein intake to protect muscle mass and to help people feel full.

It is worth noting that some groups of people require a more restrictive version of the ketogenic diet in order to produce a high level of ketone bodies to manage their conditions, e.g., children with epilepsy. This group may require more careful monitoring to make sure nutritional intake is sufficient.

9.5.8 ARE GRAINS, BEANS, LEGUMES, AND FRUITS ESSENTIAL FOR HEALTH?

The ketogenic diet is often criticised for excluding whole grains, beans, legumes, and fruits, which are promoted as being important for health. Another consideration is that humans evolved without these foods, and some individuals cannot tolerate them without discomfort and digestive issues.

The ketogenic diet also avoids most high-sugar fruits, such as grapes, bananas, mangos, and pineapples. While fruits contain various nutrients and dietary fibre, most vegetables offer comparable nutrition without the carbohydrates and sugars that can interfere with ketosis.

Diets containing animal-sourced foods are high in nutrient

density, which is a common feature of well-formulated ketogenic diets, ensuring that nutritional goals can be achieved.

9.5.9 WHAT ABOUT THE MICROBIOME?

A healthy microbiome influenced by various factors like diet, exercise, stress, geography, and medications is difficult to define. The balance of bacterial types and species diversity appears to be important, and this may be achieved with a variety of whole-food eating patterns. Processed foods appear detrimental to the microbiome, disrupting the balance of various bacterial species. There are metabolic differences in a higher carbohydrate versus lower carbohydrate diet that can produce differences in the microbiome that may be healthy in the context of the different dietary choices. A well-formulated ketogenic diet using whole foods has been shown to positively influence the microbiome, which has been reported to contribute to the success of this approach in some conditions.[21]

9.5.10 DOES THE KETOGENIC DIET CAUSE CRAVINGS OR DISORDERED EATING?

A ketogenic diet is a sustainable and effective method for achieving health and weight loss goals. It involves significant changes to an existing meal plan, restricting what may be perceived as pleasure and comfort foods such as chips, confectionery, chocolate, ice cream, fast foods, and soda. This can cause temporary cravings as the body adjusts and hormone signalling normalises.

Carbohydrate reduction helps stabilise blood sugar levels, preventing rapid blood sugar spikes and crashes, which are among the most common causes of food cravings, especially for high-sugar and carbohydrate-heavy foods. A ketogenic diet allows for various nutritious and satisfying foods, including meats, fish, eggs, nuts, seeds, full-fat dairy, non-starchy vegetables, and healthy fats like avocados and olive oil. With some planning, enjoying delicious meals while maintaining ketosis is not only achievable but may be more enjoyable than many other weight-loss programs that use low-fat or point systems.

Some people struggle with their relationship with food, especially ultra-processed foods, and demonstrate addictive behaviours towards these types of foods. As many as 20% of adults may meet the criteria for this condition, which may be rooted in childhood trauma or other neurobiological vulnerabilities. Clinicians have begun to recognise that this population needs more support to be successful in sticking to dietary changes, and some have developed special programs to assist these individuals.[2]

In conclusion, a ketogenic diet may be adapted to meet health goals that could include gaining, losing, or maintaining body weight while benefiting from the therapeutic effects of nutritional ketosis.

9.5.11 DOES THE KETOGENIC DIET AFFECT BONE HEALTH?

Studies involving children with severe epilepsy may drive concerns about the potential harm of the ketogenic diet on bone health. In this population, which often has multiple challenges, the combination of a ketogenic diet and metabolic differences may create an environment where bone health could be compromised. Medication effects and physical limitations may also contribute to this. It is important to note that these findings are specific to children with epilepsy and should not be applied to the general population. Long-term results have shown the ketogenic diet to be safe for epilepsy treatment, but it is crucial to ensure proper surveillance, correct ratios, and nutritional sufficiency in children and adolescents to ensure growth trajectories.[2]

Long-term adherence to the ketogenic diet does not appear to be linked to poor bone health; in fact, metabolic conditions like type 2 diabetes and insulin resistance can contribute to osteoporosis. Rather, avoiding the foods that may cause these conditions, such as soft drinks, fried foods, processed foods, sugary foods, and refined grains, would be beneficial.

9.5.12 WILL THE KETOGENIC DIET DAMAGE YOUR KIDNEYS?

The ketogenic diet is often misunderstood as a high-protein diet, which has promoted confusion around potential effects on the kidneys. In fact, the ketogenic diet is moderate in protein content, which is in common with other dietary patterns. As obesity, insulin resistance, and diabetes are the primary contributors to kidney dysfunction, it makes sense that the ketogenic diet could provide benefits for this population. Studies have found this approach improves kidney function in individuals with diabetes-related kidney disease, obesity, and polycystic kidney disease, and it has not been found to have a negative effect on kidney function.[22]

The risk of kidney stones is low for most individuals on a ketogenic diet. Individuals with obesity and chronic kidney disease, regardless of dietary choices, are most at risk of kidney stones. Genetic factors may also contribute to the risk. The benefits of reducing risk factors like obesity and type 2 diabetes should be weighed against other risks, as kidney disease generally improves with a ketogenic diet. Seeking the support of an experienced practitioner is recommended for further guidance.

9.5.13 DOES A KETOGENIC DIET INCREASE THE RISK OF GALLBLADDER DISEASE?

Metabolic disease is strongly linked to gallbladder disease, with abnormalities in lipid metabolism contributing to the risk. These abnormalities, such as low HDL-c and high triglycerides, promote cholesterol crystal formation, leading to gallstone formation. A reduced carbohydrate diet can improve metabolic health and increase HDL-c, supporting bile acid flow and reducing gallstone disease risk.

In a low-fat diet context, rapid weight loss can increase the risk of gallstones, but using a higher-fat approach during weight loss can prevent their development. Seeking support from an experienced practitioner and a slow transition to a ketogenic diet may be appropriate if you have a history of gallbladder disease. In the same way, if you have had your gallbladder removed, a slow transition to a low-carbohydrate or ketogenic approach is recommended.[23]

9.5.14 Can a ketogenic diet trigger a gout attack?

Gout flares are linked to metabolic dysfunction and inflammation, a condition that has significantly increased in the last 20 years. Consumption of sugar-sweetened beverages may increase fructose in the diet, leading to elevated uric acid levels. Lowering carbohydrates in the diet can lower uric acid production and address insulin resistance and inflammation.[12]

Ketone body metabolism creates competition for the uric acid excretion pathway that can result in temporary increases in uric acid concentrations as the body adapts to nutritional ketosis.[22] An experienced practitioner can advise on individual risk and recommend a temporary treatment plan. Reducing carbohydrate content in the diet slowly at first may be beneficial as it allows more time for the body to adapt. Consistency in following a ketogenic approach is recommended to avoid readaptation challenges.

9.5.15 Does the ketogenic diet increase your risk of chronic diseases?

Concerns about increased risk of chronic disease when using a ketogenic diet are generally related to the higher fat content and the assumption that this causes poor metabolic health. The confusion is rooted in studies labelling diets as 'high-fat', which are often high in carbohydrates and usually contain processed foods. Scientific evidence consistently confirms that a properly formulated ketogenic diet is safe, beneficial for obesity and diabetes, and can help with chronic health conditions like cardiovascular disease, neurodegenerative diseases, cognitive decline, fatty liver disease, chronic inflammatory conditions, sleep disorders, and mental health conditions.[12]

9.5.16 Is a ketogenic diet good for long-term health?

The ketogenic diet has been criticised for its lack of long-term data, suggesting it should only be used for short-term weight loss. However, studies in patients with type 2 diabetes and a UK GP practice have shown positive results when maintaining nutritional ketosis over a number of years. A recent study of healthy women who reported sustained ketosis for nearly 4 years showed no adverse effects, and results suggest that this metabolic state is protective against insulin resistance while preserving metabolic flexibility.[2]

In a time when 93% of the US population has poor metabolic health and over 70% of food consumption comes from foods absent from preagricultural diets, adopting a more ancestral way of eating seems like an excellent choice.

9.5.17 Is a ketogenic diet affordable and sustainable?

The affordability of a low-carbohydrate or ketogenic diet is a common question raised when considering sustainability. Studies show that a well-formulated ketogenic diet is nutrient-dense and cost-effective, with savings from fewer meals, snacks, medications, and clinic visits. This approach has been successful in low-resource settings in South Africa and India.[2]

Many individuals who have achieved their health goals using a ketogenic diet find the benefits outweigh any perceived downsides. Long-term ketogenic diets have been used with success in type 1 diabetes, mental health conditions, healthy females, and a metabolically healthy mixed population.[2] These data suggest that a ketogenic lifestyle may be sustained in the long term for those experiencing benefits and who are committed to the approach. Individuals who struggle with the symptoms of carbohydrate or processed food addiction may need additional support from a professional as well as family and community support.

9.6 Getting started with a ketogenic diet

Before embarking on a ketogenic diet, it is advisable to speak to your doctor. This is especially important if you have any medical conditions or you are taking medication. A doctor or other healthcare professional who is experienced in ketogenic therapies may be able to provide additional support. People on medication like insulin or other medication to control blood glucose or blood pressure will need to work with their doctor as the medication may need to be reduced or otherwise adjusted. This is also important for those on medication for mental health conditions who will need to work with their medical team.

In basic terms, a well-formulated ketogenic diet focuses on sufficient protein (minimum of around 1.5 g per kg lean body mass or goal) combined with non-starchy vegetables, leafy greens, and natural fats found in whole foods, dairy, rendered fats, or minimally processed cold-pressed oils. You are aiming to keep carbohydrates below 50 g/day, or, for some people, staying below 30 g/day works best. Keeping away from foods in packets or foods with lists of ingredients avoids many of the problems that come with navigating our food environment. In the same way, products advertised as 'keto-friendly' can be problematic for some, and the labelling may require careful examination.

A simple approach is to choose your protein, add vegetables and/or leafy greens, and consider whether additional fat may be required for flavour or satiety. Look at substitutes for foods like rice and pasta; cauliflower rice or courgette ribbons can be used instead.

If your goal is weight loss, remember you will be burning your own fat stores initially. As you continue your journey, the fat intake from your food may need to be adjusted upwards in order to maintain weight.

The table below gives a basic framework of foods to consider or avoid. Foods in packets or bottles tend to have hidden sugars and starches.

Unlimited	Be mindful*	Avoid	Fats for cooking or flavour
All meat types: Beef, lamb, pork, chicken, venison, buck, ostrich Other: bacon, sausage, ham, bone marrow Organ meats (offal): liver, brain, chicken feet, chicken heart, tripe, etc. Cultural variants: dried meat, e.g. jerky or droëwors (without sugar), pepperoni, salami, chorizo **Fish** All fish (also canned) Consider including fatty fish for omega 3, e.g. salmon, mackerel, anchovies, sardines, and herring	Dairy (full-fat, no added sugar) Cheese, cream cheese, cottage cheese, cream, Greek yoghurt, maas (sour milk), kefir, soft cheeses, etc. **Non-starchy vegetables** Cauliflower, broccoli, mushrooms, peppers, celery, baby marrow, aubergine	**All sugars** Syrups, honey, maple syrup, condensed milk, coconut sugar, dextrose, maltose, etc. **Grains/starchy/flour products** All bread, wraps, lentils, beans, pasta, rice, rice cakes, couscous noodles, cereals, oats, oatmeal, biscuits, puddings, corn flour, tapioca flour, etc. **Processed foods and high-sugar snacks** Crisps, chips, chocolate, ice cream, dried fruit, fast-foods, pizza, custard, condensed milk, etc.	Butter Ghee Tallow and lard (all rendered fats) Coconut oil

Unlimited	Be mindful*	Avoid	Fats for cooking or flavour
Shellfish Oysters, crab, calamari, prawns **Eggs** All types **Leafy greens** Lettuce, spinach, kale, cabbage, collards, seaweed, rocket, etc.	**Tree nuts** Macadamia, Brazil, almonds, hazelnuts, etc. **Low-sugar fruits** Avocado, cucumber, tomatoes, strawberries, blueberries, other berries	**Sugar-sweetened beverages and fruit juices** Energy drinks, cordials, etc. **Starchy vegetables** Potatoes, parsnips, butternut, carrots, sweetcorn etc. **Sauces** Tomato, barbeque, marinades, mustard, peri-peri, sweet-chilli, cooking and packet sauces, dressings **Processed seed oils** Canola, sunflower, margarine	Olive oil Macadamia nut oil Avocado oil

This list contains some carbohydrates or salt/fat combinations that may be easy to overeat (individualise to goals)

Following a ketogenic diet does not necessarily require any special apps, tracking, or additional measurements (like ketones), but some people find this helpful for troubleshooting. As with any eating pattern, responses are highly individual. Additional measures or professional support may be helpful in order to achieve health goals. This may include tracking blood glucose, ketones, and dietary intake. A food diary can help identify problem foods. Noting how you feel after certain meals can help you identify sensitivities or foods that trigger changes in mood or affect gut health.

For further information, see Resources (at the back of the book).

9.6.1 Common symptoms during adaptation and 'keto flu'

Keto flu is a term used to describe common symptoms experienced during the adaptation to a ketogenic diet that can include fatigue, headaches, muscle cramps, mild constipation, and lightheadedness. These symptoms normally resolve quickly and occur due to the reduction in carbohydrates, which alters signalling pathways, causing the body to release water and sodium. This is caused by a lower carbohydrate intake, where the body uses up glycogen stores and insulin levels fall, leading to a diuretic effect. The lowering of insulin is one of the desired effects that promotes a state of fat burning.

An effective remedy is to increase fluid intake with 1/2-1 teaspoon of salt (1–2 g sodium) daily, which can be consumed via bone broth or bouillon. Some individuals may benefit from additional salt on an ongoing basis, but a personalised approach is important. Muscular symptoms can be supported by adding elemental magnesium (200–400 mg/day) to the fluid and salt routine. Potassium intake may also be considered if there are ongoing muscle symptoms, but ensuring sufficient salt intake usually prevents this. Ongoing symptoms require clinical assessment and review of nutritional intake in case there are other medical factors to consider. For most people, this stage passes quickly, within 7–10 days.[12,24]

9.7 Conclusion

A well-formulated ketogenic diet that focuses on whole foods is a way of eating that aligns closely with ancestral eating patterns where populations appeared to be largely free from the burden of chronic disease we are experiencing today. The modern food environment, along with other lifestyle factors, has contributed to an epidemic of poor metabolic health and chronic disease. Reducing carbohydrates in the diet can improve metabolic health via various pathways, and a ketogenic diet amplifies the effects by promoting nutritional ketosis and the production of ketone bodies. This metabolic state offers additional benefits, particularly for those with severe metabolic disease, neurological conditions, and mental health conditions.

Misconceptions and misunderstandings around the ketogenic diet are common, but a critical look at the evidence suggests that concerns are largely unfounded. A reduced-carbohydrate, ketogenic way of eating has been proven to address insulin resistance, type 2 diabetes, and obesity – major risk factors for heart disease and cancer.

An individualised approach is one of the key components of a successful implementation, and this should be tailored to individual health goals. Appropriate medical monitoring is advised, especially where medications are in use and adjustments may be required. A growing body of medical practitioners is recognising the importance of metabolic health and the potential applications of the ketogenic diet for a variety of conditions. Momentum is gathering and new research appears on a monthly basis, so we can be confident the future is looking bright for personalised reduced carbohydrate approaches in healthcare.

IMPORTANT: I want to mention here that if you are thinking about trying the ketogenic diet and you're on medications, you will need to find a doctor who knows what they are doing to help you titrate off those medications. The shift in your body's metabolism happens so quickly when you remove sugar and carbohydrates that taking certain medications on the ketogenic diet can be dangerous.

CHAPTER 10

EXERCISE

If you just diet and don't incorporate those other factors that influence overall metabolic health, you may not be as successful as you might otherwise be. In other words, you won't be truly metabolically healthy. You'd probably be a lot healthier than you were, but not necessarily as healthy as you could be if you incorporated these other things into your life. Exercise is probably the next big thing. The others that come to mind are sleep, and trying to reduce, or at least manage, the stress in your life.

I talked a bit earlier about Dr Ben Bocchicchio, who has a double PhD in exercise physiology and health and physical education. He has been talking about his exercise program for 50 years. He's trained a ton of regular folks just like you and me, but also a lot of really prominent, famous people who he has been able to help as well. He speaks about it in a book that he's written called *15 Minutes to Fitness*,[25] where his concept is that a 15-minute workout twice a week is optimal, as long as you do it right.

He says that it's really, really important that you only do it twice a week. 3 days seems to be the optimal amount of recovery one needs between workouts. If you are able to work on different days all through the week on an ongoing basis, you could probably do it every three days, but for most people, the routine of doing two specific days each week seems to work best.

It's critical that you have that recovery time because, in his protocol, you're pushing your muscles to failure, and when you do that, it requires a certain amount of time for them to properly recover from that. If you don't rest, if you continue, if you go back the next day and do it again, and the next day and do it again – over time, you're going to become injured and do damage to yourself.

If you go to the gym and chat with the people working out, if they are honest, most are working with an injury of some kind. Dr Ben prides himself in the fact that all the people he's worked with have never been injured (at least not the people who listen to him and do the exercises correctly). There are two reasons for that:

1. His program is called SMaRT™ (Slow Maximum Resistance Training). When you start loading up to get the weight moving, you don't want to put stress on the ligaments and tendons. So you start very slowly and load the muscle and ligaments gradually.
2. When you finish the workout, you give yourself three days at least to recover before the next one. Your body properly recovers from that and doesn't end up breaking down, and you don't develop an injury. It's like a rechargeable battery; if you don't fully recharge it each time, it degrades and can hold less and less charge. Eventually, it's totally dead!

The concept is that you do one exercise for each major muscle group and choose a weight where you will fail totally within a window of between 30 and 90 seconds.

If you're still doing reps after 90 seconds, then next time you need to increase the weight so that you fail in that window. If you can't even get the second or third rep out and it's not even 30 seconds yet, then you need to go down in weight so that you can get back into that window. Literally, you go from one exercise to the next, and before you know it, 15 minutes are up, and you're finished.

This is what Ben says about exercise, '*I distinguish between Exercise and Activity. Exercise is a formal, structured system of muscle movements designed for a specific purpose. High-intensity exercise depends upon the muscle fibers that are recruited at the highest level carried on to muscle failure in a brief period of time (usually 30-90 seconds). High-intensity exercise should be performed infrequently (twice a week) to allow for full recovery. Activity (physical) is best suggested on a daily basis and is less structured. It can be casual, recreational or engaging in some sport activity. Its main function is to offset modern sedentary behavior. It is usually a less intrusive, steady-state exposure than high-intensity exercise.*'

The most amazing thing is that pretty much anybody can find 15 minutes twice a week to work out. The next most amazing thing is how quickly you seem to recover. I mentioned back in Chapter 7 that after the martial arts workouts, I would bounce out of bed the next day and be happy to go for a run. So the diet itself promotes really good recovery as well. When I finish this workout, I'm exhausted, but 15 minutes later, I can get up and go back to my desk and carry on working. It's like it never even happened.

In the beginning, when I first started doing these workouts, I really did notice a little bit of stiffness the next day. But after two weeks, which is really only four workouts, I was not having any feelings of stiffness at all. I literally work out, and a few minutes later, I'm good to go and carry on with my day.

It's pretty cool. I don't know if I mentioned it earlier, but when I started doing this workout, I was trying it myself and I didn't really notice any changes or benefits. Then I ended up meeting with Dr Ben at his place in Coronado, where he stays for a couple of months a year in the summer. He has a gym there, so we went and worked out, and he went through his program with me. It was only then that I realised for the first time what failure really was. It's not just thinking,

Eh, I'm tired now. It's when you totally put your mind to it and try your absolute hardest and your muscles literally cannot do anymore. And when I started doing it like that, everything changed.

We did that watershed workout in the morning and then, in the afternoon, we attended a local San Diego event organised by Jeff Kotterman from *The TriSystem Health Network*. When we arrived at the event, there was this DEXA scan truck there that does a full body composition scan and gives you readings of your bone density and muscle mass, including all your ratios of muscle and fat tissue in your body. So I went and had a DEXA scan.

About three months later, I did a scan again. I had put on four pounds of muscle mass and reduced my fat mass by another pound. I had not changed anything in the way I was eating, and I wasn't pounding protein like the bodybuilders do to try and put on weight. I really genuinely felt stronger than I've pretty much felt in my whole life. I was 54 at that time, 55 maybe. It was just incredible.

When Ben has spoken at our events, he talks about studies that show that an increase in muscle mass actually leads to a longer life. It basically adds to one's longevity. It's all very well living to 100, but you have to be all there, be strong, be able to move, play with the kids, get up and down, move things around, do the things you love, not only walk and climb up stairs, but maybe even take a hike or go on a bike ride, you have to be able to have conversations with people, you have to have some quality of life. I believe that this is what is in store for me in my old age – that when I reach those later years – I won't be a burden on society. I'll still be a functioning person who can have a real conversation with someone. I'm confident that my quality of life will be a lot better than it would have been if I didn't do this.

Going back to Dr Ben's protocol, I think you just need to go back to the Paleolithic days to see the wisdom in it. People didn't eat a lot of carbohydrates. They were primarily hunters. The women and children did gather some nuts and berries when they were in season, but mainly, they all ate a lot of meat and fat. Some of them even drank the blood. They were active, too, especially the hunters who had to go long distances and run a lot, but now and again, they would end up doing something hard which would really tax their muscles completely. I think that's what this exercise program mimics.

Mark Sisson talks about it a lot as well. Mark has written a bunch of books about the paleo and ketogenic diets, and he started an organisation called Primal Kitchen. He's always talking about exercise and pretty much says we should all strive to be active each day, and on the odd occasion, we need to lift something heavy.

Dr Ben talks about the different muscle fibres that come into use progressively. There are types I, IIa, and IIb. As each one gets to failure, the next set of muscle fibres are engaged, and you have to exhaust all of them to reach a critical threshold. Then, if you get to the IIb fibres and you take them to failure, your muscles *adapt upwardly* to compensate so that they can manage the stress better next time. That's where the increase in muscle mass comes from, which is really interesting.

CHAPTER 11

HISTORICAL FACTORS, CORPORATE MANIPULATION, AND THE CHEMISTRY OF ADDICTION

Continuing with the Paleolithic theme a bit more, your body knows what it actually needs, although there is one caveat to that. These days, we are just absolutely bombarded with advertising and propaganda from organisations that have a vested interest in the status quo, in us continuing to eat all this rubbish, and as much of it as we do – mainly the sugar industry, the wheat and corn industries, and the pharmaceutical industry. This and the pathetically flawed US Dietary Guidelines and all the misinformation that we are bombarded with on a daily basis can all be linked back, pretty much, to an epidemiologist called Ancel Keys. He believed that saturated fat in the diet was the cause of *degenerative heart disease, which was defined as coronary disease, angina pectoris, infarction, chronic myocarditis and myocardial degeneration.* He set out to prove it, and in 1953 he published a paper where he had plotted the data of six countries comparing saturated fat consumption against death from degenerative heart disease. The dots fit almost perfectly on an exponential graph showing ever-increasing deaths as saturated fat in the diet rose. His paper concluded, *'Whether or not cholesterol, etc., are involved, it must be concluded that dietary fat somehow is associated with cardiac diseases mortality,* and this became known as the *Diet-Heart-Hypothesis.'*

He bullied it through and was very involved in beating down John Yudkin's opposing hypothesis that sugar was actually to blame. This ushered in the low-fat era. Margarine replaced butter, seed oils replaced lard and butter for cooking and the dogmatic nutritional advice that pervades our society today came to be. Everything that we've been brought up to believe about what is healthy can basically be traced back to that paper.

There are two critical issues to note here. The first has to do with a fundamental flaw in any epidemiological study. *Association does not prove causation.* For example, a problem raised by Jeff Nobbs in his article, 'The Problem with Observational Studies (Epidemiology)' states the following: *'Study Shows People Who Brush Teeth Less Frequently Are at Higher Risk for Heart Disease.'* The problem is, we don't know whether teeth brushing is actually the thing preventing heart disease, or if people who have good oral hygiene happen to have healthier lifestyle habits in general.

The second, and most egregious issue, however, is that his paper was totally fraudulent and in academic circles it is referred to as scientific misconduct. The original data set was made up of 22 countries, not 6, and when you plot the other 16 points on the graph there is no apparent association at all, no exponential curve, just a random scatter pattern of dots. There wasn't even any association in the first place, let alone a causal factor of any kind.

Talking of outside influences, Belinda Fettke has done a whole lot of incredible research and exposed the sinister role of the 7th Day Adventist Church in demonising meat and advancing the narrative of Veganism. I hope that she is able to publish all these findings in a book soon.

Ok, so there's more than one caveat. There is another sinister force at play here which most people are not aware of. One of the really interesting things about all high-carb, ultra-processed food companies is that a lot of them are now owned by the cigarette companies. We're all aware that a little while back, cigarette smoking started to become taboo. More and more people were quitting, and their sales were hurting badly, so they all put their heads together and said, 'What are we going to do about this?' One of the things that they were experts at was cultivating an addiction. So they looked at how they could put that experience to work. They came up with the concept of using processed food. They bought up a bunch of these processed food companies, and they all have actual engineers in their laboratories whose job it is to work out exactly the balance of vegetable oils and sugar and a little bit of salt etc. that is required to create what they call the 'bliss point', where it triggers all of pathways in your brain that effectively elicit an addiction.

I've talked about it earlier. Carbohydrate and sugar addiction is a huge thing. A lot of that has to do with the way that these ultra-processed foods are actually created. Then these companies get into the stores and they encourage the store owners in some way to place the cereal boxes and other processed food items on the lower shelves. Someone recently explained to me that the reason for this is not arbitrary, it's eye level for the kids. The kids see these pretty boxes and chuck them into mom's shopping trolley to be taken home and consumed. It's a huge tidal wave that people are struggling against the whole time without even really realising that they're being manipulated.

That's aside from the physiological effects of consuming all of these carbohydrates, right? If you consume carbohydrates, your blood sugar skyrockets. And that triggers a response from your pancreas to release insulin. The insulin brings the blood sugar levels down, but there's now an overreaction, and the blood sugar goes really low, and you become hypoglycaemic.

That can actually be life-threatening. Your body then triggers hormones to stimulate cravings. Suddenly, you're starving, and you're literally going to kill someone (you're hangry!) if you can't get something to eat. Obviously, it's going to be all carbohydrate-centric, because that's the food that you've been told you should be eating, so then you get this huge spike again (hyperglycaemia).

Throughout the day, you're on this massive roller coaster. Your body is generating hormones to make you really hungry. This is so that you eat in order to save your life and don't go hypoglycaemic and actually have a fatal situation. On top of all of these actual blood sugar fluctuations that you're going through, the food itself that you're now consuming is addictive. You become totally addicted to these foods as well – it's a double whammy!

So, there *was* more than one caveat, this is the third. For most of us in modern society, our metabolisms are so broken that our body knowing what it actually needs is not really true anymore. Most of us eat such rubbish all our lives, and we're so used to eating so much – just look at the volume of food on our plates – it's hard to fix that. It's like you look at the plate of nutrient-dense food, and it doesn't look like nearly enough food. If you don't see that volume on your plate, you think that you're not eating enough, and you think you must still be hungry.

One of the things Dr Rob Cywes talks about with his patients when he's helping them with strategies to cope with carb and sugar addiction is that they need to eat sequentially. Put all the food in the middle of the table, get yourself a side plate and dish yourself some food onto that side plate and eat it. When you're finished, sit for a minute and then ask yourself, *am I genuinely still hungry?* And if you are, by all means, take some more food onto your plate and eat it. But a lot of the time, you will think, *No, you know what? I'm okay. I've eaten enough.* These days I eat off a side plate all the time, I don't even need a plate of extra food in the middle of the table, just in case. Later, you will think, *I'm so glad I didn't stuff all of that other food in my face.* That's why Rob is taking people and trying to teach them to reset their brains. He wants them to start to go back to their natural ability to monitor what they are eating, and dictate how much of it they consume.

CHAPTER 12

THE SMHP

Late in 2018, I was invited to be part of a documentary called *Fat Fiction*, but the truth of the story is that I kind of invited myself. Basically, this amazing couple had decided to make a documentary and one of the people who they chose to incorporate into it was Dr Brian Lenzkes, who I mentioned earlier in this book and with whom we are great friends.. They came out to San Diego and did a bunch of filming with him and some of his patients.

Before they came, though, he wrote to me – I was in Australia, visiting with my family and with Gary and Belinda Fettke – *'Dude, this film company has basically approached me to see if I will be part of their documentary. I have no idea who they are, what they do, or what they're about. What do you think? Should I do it?'*

I did a bunch of research and found out who they were and what they were doing. Turns out it was Jen Isenhart and Tom Hadzor from Wide Eye Productions and they were totally legit, so I told him that he should go for it.

They came out to San Diego and did a bunch of filming with him but then they went back to where they were based in Boise, Idaho. I was in Australia while they were in San Diego so when I got back, I wrote to them. At that point, we were a week away from our event in Seattle.

It was at that event that we planned to announce the launch of our clinical guidelines. I said to them, *'I don't need to be in the film, but you need to get something in there about these new clinical guidelines we're about to publish.'* I explained what they were all about.

They replied, *'Yeah, we agree, but we literally funded this thing ourselves, and we have no more money.'* So I used my points to get a flight and a hotel, and I flew out to Boise. I spent an incredible day with the two of them. We ended up doing a bunch of filming. They interviewed me in their lounge that they had turned into a studio and took me out into the hills and filmed me running up and down through the trails and built all of that into the documentary.

But for me, the biggest thing was that I got to talk about the clinical guidelines and how important they were.

Back at the beginning of 2018, I approached Gary Taubes to speak again at the San Diego event that year. He suggested to me that we do a focus group-type session where practitioners who were actually trying to embrace this concept with their patients could come up to the mic, and they could talk about what they'd been doing and the successes and failures they'd experienced. Gary was writing his next book on the subject, so it would have provided some great feedback and content for him. For me, it was good because it was another session in which Gary would be on stage. He is a big draw.

He suggested to me that I contact a lady named Adele Hite. She was a Registered Dietitian (RD), and he'd obviously been speaking with her a lot. He won't take credit for it, but I believe that in his mind he was thinking, *I need to put Doug in contact with Adele because great things might come of that.* He introduced me to her and suggested I should get her to moderate this discussion. I wrote to her and asked if she would do it.

She replied to me with a two-page email that was just like a total brain dump of everything she had in her mind. She really wanted Therapeutic Carbohydrate Reduction (TCR) to be considered Standard of Care (SoC). The thing I loved about her was that she was not combative. She didn't want to point fingers and say, 'You're wrong,' and 'We're right,' She just wanted to put forward an alternative to the current SoC. If people stop consuming excessive carbohydrates, their metabolism changes completely at that point, and her thought was that the current SoC often didn't apply.

She told me that she had been on the jury in a malpractice trial, and the judge had to explain to them what 'Standard of Care' was so that they could understand whether or not this physician was guilty of malpractice. The actual legal definition of SoC was in her email to me and I put it up on a slide for most of my opening talks at all these events I've done since.

> *'Standard of Care' is defined as 'providing health care in accordance with the standards of practice among members of the same health care profession with similar training and experience and situated in the same or similar communities at the time the health care is rendered.' In other words, SoC does not come from what is taught in professional training, from public health policy, or even from clinical care guidelines, although these can inform and help define a Standard of Care. Rather, Standard of Care comes from what a community of clinicians **do** in the actual provision of care.*

I remember when she first sent this email to me, it was like her vision was just so enormous that I literally went weak at the knees. I was thinking, *I just asked you if you would moderate a discussion at our event with practitioners who are doing this in their practice.*

But as time went on, I read it over and over and over again. And the more I read it, and especially the more I read this definition, it started to occur to me that we actually had so many building blocks in place already.

Establishing a community was well underway and we were creating more and more training to teach any of these physicians and practitioners who were interested in learning about it. We had tons of doctors and practitioners who now would be prepared to put their name to something that said, *'Under these conditions, and in the absence of carbohydrates, this is actually the preferred course of action.'* Effectively, over time, that establishes Standard of Care. It's a consensus amongst this community of practitioners who now have the training and who all practice TCR.

I got back to her, and I said, *'You know, I feel like maybe we can do something here.'*

She came to the event and moderated that session but as soon as she went home, we started working. She felt the best way to start this was to actually develop a clinical guidelines document. Even though the legal definition says they are not in and of themselves Standard of Care, they can greatly support the discussions around TCR that eventually end up in a consensus which establishes Standard of Care.

She started to write the document and we realised that we needed a panel of advisors to bounce this off. So I got 15 practitioners, really, really prominent people, Tim Noakes and Gary Fettke and David Unwin from the UK, who's huge in this space, and Eric Westman and Will Yancey and 11 others. There were just so many really experienced practitioners who all agreed to be on this panel.

Adele basically kicked me out of the kitchen at that point. She said, 'You're not a clinician, so you can't contribute to this.' All I did was take roadblocks out of their way and facilitate these discussions and meetings.

Then she just bounced this manuscript off the panel over and over until, finally, there was a consensus that it was ready to go. They reached this consensus just before our 2019 Seattle event. We put it on the LowCarb*USA* site because that was all we had at the time. It got a lot of traffic when we published it there, but it wasn't an ideal place for it.

We got a ton of people giving really good feedback about it. We kind of knew that it was something that was needed, but it definitely wasn't yet in the right place. I also realised that it would be important to have some kind of community for these practitioners to be able to talk about things and establish that consensus.

On LowCarb*USA*, I had started this concept of professional communities, and I was trying to get these practitioners to join up and become a part of it. I got a handful, maybe 20 people signed up, so it really wasn't getting any traction.

Then, in 2020, when we were in Boca for our event in January, Dr Tro Kalayjian, from the *LowCarbMD Podcast,* was one of our speakers. Apparently – I only became aware of this much later – he had a discussion with Pam and basically said to her that we need to have an organisation that represents all of the practitioners in this space, just like the AMA (American Medical Association) and OMA (Obesity Medicine Association). We need to have something that supports us, understands us, and can have our backs. He said to her, 'I think Doug should do it.'

Maybe I'm glad that I didn't hear it at the time because it probably would have overwhelmed me a little with everything else I had going on at the event. A month later or so, sometime in February, I saw a tweet from him, basically saying that we need to have an organisation like this.

I had no idea at that stage that this other conversation had happened in Boca. I wrote to him and said, 'I already have these organisations on LowCarb*USA*, but we got zero traction from it. How are we going to do this?' We talked about it backwards and forwards and ended up agreeing that what we needed was a proper non-profit organisation that would represent all practitioners in this space.

I put a board together, and we started talking about what we wanted to do, and in the meantime, I was learning how to create a non-profit. It was a lot of learning and a lot of paperwork to do, which I hate. If you're not going to pay a lawyer a ton of money to do this for you, it is a mission.

Then, just at that time, COVID shut everything down.

What made it even more difficult was that the government was shut down while we were trying to apply for, and establish, a non-profit organisation. Initially, the employees weren't even there; it was simply shut down. Then, they started to get some of those employees to work from home.

Amazingly enough, though it was slow, I actually made progress. Towards the end of that year, the non-profit was in place. In the meantime, we were trying to decide what it was going to do and what the website was going to look like.

We had already been going backwards and forwards about a name for the organisation. Dr Eric Westman was the one who eventually came up with the name *Society of Metabolic Health Practitioners*. We wanted to move away from the terms low-carb or ketogenic, as those can be very polarising, and just talk about metabolic health, since anything that can contribute to metabolic health needs to be a part of this conversation.

So the Society of Metabolic Health Practitioners (SMHP™) was born. But what is metabolic health, actually? There's not any formal definition of it that I know of, but essentially, it's where all the body processes are functioning within a range that doesn't place excessive stress on the system and is largely related to how your body processes food and creates and uses energy. A kind of homeostatic green zone, as it were, where the harmful byproducts of metabolism are minimal and easily processed without harm, repair systems are functioning optimally and cellular metabolism and energetics are optimal.

We decided that we needed to migrate the clinical guidelines across to this new site so that now it would have a perfect new home, which was brilliant. Sadly, we lost Adele to a long fight with cancer, but not before she got to witness this happen, which made her *so* proud. She left a huge hole that we struggle to fill to this day.

We also had a search engine on LowCarb*USA* for people to try and find a doctor or practitioner who was sympathetic to this intervention or at least open to the concept and prepared to support the patient wanting to try TCR. So, we moved that onto the SMHP site as well.

There were a few other things we had started to create on LowCarb*USA*, like this little database of great scientific papers that explored the efficacy of TCR. By this time we had become aware of the database of papers Sarah Rice had created so, instead of reinventing the wheel, we just put a link in straight to her database and didn't try to do anything clever ourselves because it would have been a complete waste of time.

We introduced this concept of having grand rounds once a month, where our practitioners and our scientists can educate our members on interesting or cutting edge concepts. We established a forum where people can have these discussions in order to contribute to establishing TCR as Standard of Care.

I think the most important thing that we introduced was an accreditation process because we wanted to establish legitimacy for the practitioners and a recognisable way to indicate that a practitioner met an acceptable standard of education and understanding of the TCR concepts and to provide them with credibility in the workplace and with their patients. Now an accredited SMHP member can proudly display the credential MHP (Metabolic Health Practitioner) behind their name and display the cool orange SMHP Accredited badge on their websites and in their communications.

We came up with a few different pathways that they could follow in order to achieve this accreditation. One of them was just basic training. We identified a core set of training modules, developed by the Nutrition Network, that the candidate would have to work through in order to get it done that way. There are other ways as well, including one called 'clinical practice': If they have been practising TCR for years, then they can write an essay and describe their practice and talk about some successful cases and a few difficult cases that they have had. The board decided that everybody had to at least complete the ethics course.

These different pathways are now defined, and if a practitioner submits an application and it is approved by the review board, they become an MHP. Even Brian Lenzkes is now Brian Lenzkes MD,

MHP. He is an accredited Metabolic Health Practitioner through our organisation.

We had a website designed for us that was never brilliant, but got the job done. It was like that for us for a few years but literally, at the time of writing this book, we've just gone live with a spectacular brand-new website. It now looks like a really professional organisation, which is brilliant; because that's what we are.

I'd been putting out some teasers that it was coming soon, and then we went live with the site in December 2020. Anybody can put their names in and be listed in our list of providers. However, in order to participate in the forums, grand rounds, research academy, and become accredited, they have to become members. That was what we visualised. We didn't want to rely on donations if we didn't have to, so this would hopefully be our revenue stream.

We put it out there and it just took off. I was astounded that we had, I don't know, probably 150-200 people in the first month or so already signed up as members. It didn't keep going at that rate, but it has continued to grow. We have six or seven hundred members now. We have more than 120 people accredited at this point and tons more in the pipeline somewhere along the way of getting to the point where they can submit their application.

It's been an absolute – I can't even think of the right word – it's just been extraordinary! I remember, quite near the beginning, I had written to a lady doctor who had put in her application for accreditation. We checked it out and approved her application. I sent her an email saying, *'Congratulations, you've been approved for accreditation. You can use the credentials MHP now and here's the badge that you can use on your website or your communications should you choose to. Congratulations!'*

She wrote back and said, *'You know, Doug, this means more to me than when I became an MD because now I finally feel like I'm going to be able to help people.'*

That has stayed with me. We've heard something similar many times subsequently, but that was the first time that I had heard somebody really vocalise their appreciation for what this effort has meant for the community and how much they value and treasure it. That was epic for me.

Here are a few more testimonials we've received:

After sending an approval to Keevn Ott, he wrote back and said, '*Great news. Thank you so much. What a great organisation! I truly believe in the message the SMHP promotes, and what I have learned so far has completely changed my optometry practice and how I work with patients.*'

So it's not just medical doctors; here is an optometrist who is utilising TCR to help some of his patients with their vision issues.

Even nurse practitioners and nurses, Sarah Aitken and her sister Catherine are always at our conferences; just two of the most amazing people.

Sarah says, '*Me and my sister Catherine are both excited to come back. I've just signed up for the next event, and you've done a great job with it. I have never attended a conference where I've stayed for every single speaker all the way to the end.*'

Dr Karen Jerome-Zapadka is a doctor who is on one of our committees within the SMHP, and she wrote back and said, '*I am so indebted and grateful to you both and the profound impact that LowCarbUSA and SMHP have had on my own health and life and career.*'

So as I mentioned, we've got a brand new SMHP website that we've just gone live with. It keeps growing, and every time I do an opening talk at one of the LowCarb*USA* events, I talk about the new developments since the last time, and there's always something new that I can talk about.

Since we launched the site with the bare bones, some of the new things that we've added are resources for practitioners and patients. We've got pages where practitioners and patients can go and find all these free resources to help them, created by our Resources Committee which is chaired by Dr. Jodi Nishida. These are resources that practitioners and patients can learn from and that patients can take to their doctors to educate them about TCR and hopefully encourage them to support their patients in adopting it. They can say to their doctors, 'I want to do this; you need to help me and here's information from a legitimate organisation.' We keep adding a new one every few months so that library is growing nicely.

We're always trying to encourage more and more people to put their thoughts out there in the forums so that we can establish conversations that can eventually lead to a consensus which would establish Standard of Care for Therapeutic Carbohydrate Reduction.

Back late in 2023, we launched a medical journal called the Journal of Metabolic Health (JMH). At many other journals, the reviewers are often very anti-low-carb or against the ketogenic diet or any of these metabolic therapies, and they make it really difficult or sometimes just downright impossible to get the paper published. Now we have a journal in place that does not have these biases in the review panels, so people are able to submit papers or case studies on some of their patients, and they can get it published.

Sometimes, people look at a case study and think, *That's just one person, and it's not a trial, so it doesn't count.* But if we get more and more documented n=1 cases out there, after a while, n=1 becomes n=thousands, and it becomes a tipping point. There are so many cases that show the efficacy of TCR and indicate that it at least warrants further scrutiny. Maybe it will even lead to larger cohort studies. It makes people sit up and think, *Hey, I should look at this. Maybe there's something to this. This isn't just one person talking anymore; thousands of people are saying the same thing. Maybe I need to take note, and even take it to my patients.* That's obviously first prize for us.

One of our amazing members, Dr Melanie Tidman is a professor at three different universities where she runs a journal club and teaches people how to write and submit academic papers. When she heard about us launching this journal, she came to us and said, '*Hey, I'd love to create something like this for the SMHP.*' She has created an awesome Research Academy program for us. The amount of work she's done on it is astounding. She's produced a series of ten lectures on all the different phases of this process, from the point of coming up with a concept to eventually submitting the paper, and then responding to the reviewers. She talks about how to navigate that whole process so that you can eventually get your paper published.

It's gone live now with the new website, and we just had our first live Journal Club meeting in December 2024.

The SMHP has published its first consensus paper through this journal, which marks a breakthrough in advocacy for the application of TCR for type 1 diabetes.[26] This validated approach for obtaining agreement amongst experts is another way in which the SMHP is able to support clinicians using TCR in practice. The more we get this information out there in the community, the more legitimacy we add to this whole TCR protocol.

Then, the latest thing that we've added is a growing library of recipes. Dr Tro Kalayjian, who is on our board of directors, was the main instigator behind this. His idea is that the American Diabetes Association has hundreds of recipes published on its website, and they are all full of carbs and sugar, and just rubbish. Tro wanted to provide alternative low-carb and ketogenic recipes that eliminate all the sugar and carbs. We only started with twelve recipes when it first launched, but we're going to start running competitions and get people to submit their ideas. I think, fairly quickly, that's going to grow into a really nice database of recipes. Recipes are a really good traffic generator for websites, so I'm hopeful that it will bring more traffic to our site.

I'm hoping this book will turn out to be another way to get the message out and make more people aware of the fact that we even exist.

CONCLUSION

Our society today is plagued by a number of chronic diseases that so many people suffer from. Most of these folks have a cabinet full of drugs that they need to take on a daily basis to try to manage these conditions, and their prognoses and quality of life are pretty dire in most cases. My message is that there is hope! So many of these conditions can be reversed, or at the very least managed so much more successfully, often with an elimination of most, or all, medications, just with a change in diet and lifestyle. Dare I say, they can even be preventable if these changes are adopted early on. If you're open to making these changes, it will literally change your life.

LowCarb*USA* and the SMHP are awesome places to start. We are cultivating a really beautiful community of patients and practitioners where they can come and learn, and collaborate, and find support. It is the most incredible crowd of people that I have ever come across in my life. We've never been able to really pinpoint the reasons behind this. I don't know whether it's the type of person who can wrap their head around going against the norm – against the grain, as Tim

Noakes says – and doing something different because they believe it will work, or whether it's literally the change in metabolism, the reduction in inflammation, and other physiological changes, especially in the brain, that make people more relaxed and more enjoyable to be around. If you can come to one of our events, you'll see for yourself that the environment and the atmosphere are second to none. I've often had people say to me that it's like one big family.

If you're still reading at this point, then I would like to thank you from the bottom of my heart. Hopefully, you are still here because something has resonated with you, and you want to learn more and see if you might be able to change your life, too. Maybe you're a patient with some chronic condition that you want to try to reverse and get off your medications. Maybe you're a practitioner who is sick of not being able to help your patients get better. Maybe you're just someone who wants to improve your general metabolic health and live your best life.

Scan the QR code that follows to find a list of resources on both our websites to help you on your journey of discovery and improved metabolic health. Watch all the training and testimonial videos. Check out all the resources and handouts we have. Search for a practitioner who can help you on this journey. Print out our clinical guidelines and use them in your practice or take them to your own doctor. Participate in our Grand Rounds training sessions. Learn how to turn your cases into a paper that you can publish in a journal. Become accredited so that you can go out as an MHP and practise metabolic medicine with confidence.

As for the doctors who put their heads in the sand and refuse to acknowledge any of the overwhelming evidence that is emerging, or who refuse to offer this intervention as an option to their patients, I'm not the only one who believes that's malpractice. Patient autonomy is vital. Your doctor should be laying out all the options for you, without any bias, and then allowing you – given all the information – to make a decision on your course of treatment. It's your choice!

If nothing else, what I hope you got out of this book was a sense of power to take your life back.

Scan the QR code for a list of resources:

https://bit.ly/the-road-to-metabolic-health

RESOURCES

1. **The SMHP Clinical Guidelines**

(https://thesmhp.org/clinical-guidelines/)
The Society for Metabolic Health Practitioners provides support and training for clinicians as well as general resources. Clinical guidelines can support the implementation of Therapeutic Carbohydrate Reduction (you can print a copy for your healthcare provider). Patient and clinician handouts are also available.

2. **SMHP Practitioner listing**

(https://thesmhp.org/directory/)
The SMHP has a list of practitioners who consider metabolic health and lifestyle interventions alongside the standard medical approach and are available to support you on your journey.

3. **Recommended Reading**

- Bikman B, Fung J. Why We Get Sick: The Hidden Epidemic at the Root of Most Chronic Disease——and How to Fight It. Dallas, TX: BenBella Books; 2020. 270 p.
- Bocchicchio V "Ben", Barkley C. 15 Minutes to Fitness: Dr. Ben's SMaRT Plan for Diet and Total Health. 1st edition. New York: SelectBooks; 2017. 352 p.
- Noakes TD, Murphy T, Wellington N, Kajee H, Rice SM, editors. Ketogenic: The Science of Therapeutic Carbohydrate Restriction in Human Health [Internet]. Academic Press; 2023 [cited 2023 Jul 26]. Available from: https://www.sciencedirect.com/science/article/pii/B9780182161700000218
- Phinney SD, Volek JS. The Art and Science of Low Carbohydrate Living: An Expert Guide to Making the Life-Saving Benefits of Carbohydrate Restriction Sustainable and Enjoyable. 1st edition. Lexington, KY: Beyond Obesity LLC; 2011. 316 p.
- Rice, Sarah, and Doug Reynolds. 2024. 'The Ketogenic Diet: Addressing Concerns and Considering Benefits'. LowCarb*USA*®. June 2024. https://www.lowcarbusa.org/the-ketogenic-diet/.

- Diabetes Australia. Best Practice Guidelines | Diabetes Australia [Internet]. 2019 [cited 2024 Dec 19]. Available from: https://www.diabetesaustralia.com.au/health-professional-guidelines/

REFERENCES

1. Reason S, EC W, Godfrey RJ, E M. Can a Low-Carbohydrate Diet Improve Exercise Tolerance in McArdle Disease? Journal of Rare Disorders: Diagnosis & Therapy [Internet]. 2017 Jan 1;03. Available from: https://www.researchgate.net/publication/317107130_Can_a_Low-Carbohydrate_Diet_Improve_Exercise_Tolerance_in_McArdle_Disease#fullTextFileContent

2. Rice S, Reynolds D. The Ketogenic Diet: addressing concerns and considering benefits [Internet]. LowCarbUSA®. 2024 [cited 2024 Aug 21]. Available from: https://www.lowcarbusa.org/the-ketogenic-diet/

3. Stylianou C, Kelnar C. The introduction of successful treatment of diabetes mellitus with insulin. Journal of the Royal Society of Medicine [Internet]. 2009 Jul 1 [cited 2024 Nov 19];102(7):298. Available from: https://pmc.ncbi.nlm.nih.gov/articles/PMC2711201/

4. Rollo J. Account of Two Cases of Diabetes Mellitus, with Remarks. Annals of Medicine, For the Year. [Internet]. 1797 [cited 2024 Nov 19];2:85. Available from: https://pmc.ncbi.nlm.nih.gov/articles/PMC5112440/

5. Westman EC, Yancy WS, Humphreys M. Dietary treatment of diabetes mellitus in the pre-insulin era (1914-1922). Perspect Biol Med. 2006;49(1):77–83.

6. Banting W. Letter on Corpulence, Addressed to the Public. Obesity Research [Internet]. 1993 [cited 2024 May 10];1(2):153–63. Available from: https://onlinelibrary.wiley.com/doi/abs/10.1002/j.1550-8528.1993.tb00605.x

7. Osler SW. The Principles and Practice of Medicine: Designed for the Use of Practitioners and Students of Medicine. D. Appleton; 1892. 1116 p.

8. Zinman B, Skyler JS, Riddle MC, Ferrannini E. Diabetes Research and Care Through the Ages. Diabetes Care [Internet]. 2017 Sep 12 [cited 2024 Nov 20];40(10):1302–13. Available from: https://doi.org/10.2337/dci17-0042

9. Diem P, Ducluzeau PH, Scheen A. The discovery of insulin. Diabetes Epidemiology and Management [Internet]. 2022 Jan 1 [cited 2024 Nov 18];5:100049. Available from: https://www.sciencedirect.com/science/article/pii/S2666970621000494

10. Lennerz BS, Koutnik AP, Azova S, Wolfsdorf JI, Ludwig DS. Carbohydrate restriction for diabetes: rediscovering centuries-old wisdom. J Clin Invest [Internet]. 2021 Jan 4 [cited 2021 Jan 5];131(1). Available from: https://www.jci.org/articles/view/142246

11. Wheless JW. History of the ketogenic diet. Epilepsia [Internet]. 2008 [cited 2024 Nov 18];49(s8):3–5. Available from: https://onlinelibrary.wiley.com/doi/abs/10.1111/j.1528-1167.2008.01821.x

12. Noakes TD, Murphy T, Wellington N, Kajee H, Rice SM, editors. Ketogenic: The Science of Therapeutic Carbohydrate Restriction in Human Health [Internet]. Academic Press; 2023 [cited 2023 Jul 26]. Available from: https://www.sciencedirect.com/science/article/pii/B9780128216170000218

13. Tagliabue A, Armeno M, Berk KA, Guglielmetti M, Ferraris C, Olieman J, et al. Ketogenic diet for epilepsy and obesity: Is it the same? Nutrition, Metabolism and Cardiovascular Diseases [Internet]. 2024 Jan 14 [cited 2024 Feb 13];0(0). Available from: https://www.nmcd-journal.com/article/S0939-4753(24)00016-4/fulltext

14. O'Hearn M, Lauren BN, Wong JB, Kim DD, Mozaffarian D. Trends and Disparities in Cardiometabolic Health Among US Adults, 1999-2018. Journal of the American College of Cardiology [Internet]. 2022 Jul 12 [cited 2023 Oct 30];80(2):138–51. Available from: https://www.sciencedirect.com/science/article/pii/S0735109722049944

15. Choi YJ, Jeon SM, Shin S. Impact of a Ketogenic Diet on Metabolic Parameters in Patients with Obesity or Overweight and with or without Type 2 Diabetes: A Meta-Analysis of Randomized Controlled Trials. Nutrients [Internet]. 2020 Jul [cited 2020 Jul 9];12(7):2005. Available from: https://www.mdpi.com/2072-6643/12/7/2005

16. Mujica-Parodi LR, Amgalan A, Sultan SF, Antal B, Sun X, Skiena S, et al. Diet modulates brain network stability, a biomarker for brain aging, in young adults. PNAS [Internet]. 2020 Mar 17 [cited 2020 May 19];117(11):6170–7. Available from: https://www.pnas.org/content/117/11/6170

17. Laurent N. From theory to practice: challenges and rewards of implementing ketogenic metabolic therapy in mental health. Frontiers in Nutrition [Internet]. 2024 [cited 2024 Feb 13];11. Available from: https://www.frontiersin.org/articles/10.3389/fnut.2024.1331181

18. Teicholz N. A short history of saturated fat: the making and unmaking of a scientific consensus. Current Opinion in Endocrinology, Diabetes & Obesity [Internet]. 2023 Feb [cited 2023 Jan 14];30(1):65–71.

Available from: https://journals.lww.com/10.1097/MED.0000000000000791

19. Astrup A, Magkos F, Bier DM, Brenna JT, de Oliveira Otto MC, Hill JO, et al. Saturated Fats and Health: A Reassessment and Proposal for Food-based Recommendations: JACC State-of -the-Art Review. Journal of the American College of Cardiology [Internet]. 2020 Jun 17 [cited 2020 Jun 25]; Available from: http://www.sciencedirect.com/science/article/pii/S0735109720356874

20. Zinn C, Lenferna De La Motte KA, Rush A, Johnson R. Assessing the Nutrient Status of Low Carbohydrate, High-Fat (LCHF) Meal Plans in Children: A Hypothetical Case Study Design. Nutrients [Internet]. 2022 Jan [cited 2022 Apr 13];14(8):1598. Available from: https://www.mdpi.com/2072-6643/14/8/1598

21. Allan NP, Yamamoto BY, Kunihiro BP, Nunokawa CKL, Rubas NC, Wells RK, et al. Ketogenic Diet Induced Shifts in the Gut Microbiome Associate with Changes to Inflammatory Cytokines and Brain-Related miRNAs in Children with Autism Spectrum Disorder. Nutrients [Internet]. 2024 May 7 [cited 2024 May 30];16(10):1401. Available from: https://www.ncbi.nlm.nih.gov/pmc/articles/PMC11124410/

22. Athinarayanan SJ, Roberts CGP, Vangala C, Shetty GK, McKenzie AL, Weimbs T, et al. The case for a ketogenic diet in the management of kidney disease. BMJ Open Diabetes Research and Care [Internet]. 2024 Apr 1 [cited 2024 Apr 29];12(2):e004101. Available from: https://drc.bmj.com/content/12/2/e004101

23. Cucuzzella M, Hite A, Patterson K, Heath LS& R. A clinician's guide to inpatient low carbohydrate diets for remission of type 2 diabetes: toward a standard of care protocol. Diabetes Management [Internet]. 2019 Jan 30 [cited 2019 Apr 23];9(1):7–19. Available from: https://www.openaccessjournals.com/abstract/a-clinicians-guide-to-inpatient-low-carbohydrate-diets-for-remission-of-type-2-diabetes--toward-a-standard-of-care-proto-12898.html

24. Volek JS, Kackley ML, Buga A. Nutritional Considerations During Major Weight Loss Therapy: Focus on Optimal Protein and a Low-Carbohydrate Dietary Pattern. Curr Nutr Rep [Internet]. 2024 May 30 [cited 2024 May 31]; Available from: https://doi.org/10.1007/s13668-024-00548-6

25. Bocchicchio V "Ben", Barkley C. 15 Minutes to Fitness: Dr. Ben's SMaRT Plan for Diet and Total Health. 1st edition. New York: SelectBooks; 2017. 352 p.

26. Kalayjian T, McNally BJ, Calkins MW, Cucuzzella MT, Cywes R, Dikeman H, et al. The SMHP™ position statement on therapeutic carbohydrate reduction for type 1 diabetes. Journal of Metabolic Health [Internet]. 2024 Nov 30 [cited 2024 Nov 30];7(1):9. Available from: https://journalofmetabolichealth.org/index.php/jmh/article/view/100

Printed in Great Britain
by Amazon

57477943R00092